Enhancing
THE SELF ESTEEM OF THE NURSING HOME RESIDENT

Marylou Hughes, LCSW, DPA

PROFESSIONAL PRINTING & PUBLISHING, INC.

P.O. Box 5758 · Bossier City, LA 71171-5758
318-746-6880 · 1-800-551-8783 · FAX 318-746-6995
Web Site: http://www.ppandp.com
E-mail: order@ppandp.com

ISBN 1-877735-16-7

Professional Printing & Publishing, Inc.
P.O. Box 5758
Bossier City, LA 71171-5758
318/746-6880
WATS 1-800/551-8783 - FAX 318/746-6995
Web Site: http://www.ppandp.com
E-mail: order@ppandp.com

Seventh Printing 1999

ABOUT THE AUTHOR

Dr. Marylou Hughes has been involved in the field of gerontology not only as a consultant and provider of in-service training to nursing home staff, but as a teacher, administrator, psychotherapist, and writer. She has worked with the elderly in mental health, institutional, rehabilitative, and home settings.

Included in Dr. Hughes' background are experiences in children's services, crisis intervention, and program development. For the past twenty plus years she has worked in social services as an employee of the Department of Health and Rehabilitation Services in Florida, and later in rehabilitation and mental health centers and hospitals. She is currently self-employed as a marriage counselor, psychotherapist, teacher and consultant for several private facilities in Florida.

Other books written by Dr. Hughes:
The Nursing Home and the Resident's Relatives
Mental Health Problems and the Nursing Home Resident
Revised Social Service Care Plans for Long Term Care Facilities
Restorative Approach for Nursing Home Social Workers
Social Service Policies & Procedures for LTC Facilities
Essential Psychosocial Inservices for Nursing Home Personnel
Inservices on Loss, Families, and Aging
Dying, Death, and Loss in Long Term Care
Group Psychotherapy in Long Term Care
Individual Psychotherapy in Long Term Care Settings
The Long-Term Care Family Manual

Dedicated to Alice Robinson

ACKNOWLEDGMENTS

Manuela E. Roller, Nursing Home Social Service Director

and

Vincent Cacciatore, Nursing Home Administrator

All examples are compilations rather than reports of actual events

TABLE OF CONTENTS

Chapter I

SELF ESTEEM DEFINED

If we can agree that when we feel better about ourselves we feel better about everything else, we can agree that high self esteem is an asset we want to possess. With self esteem the world is a more rewarding place in which to live.

What is this elusive quality we all strive to make our own? What is self esteem? We know esteem means to value, prize, to regard highly, and to look on with favor. With good feelings about ourselves we can manage the day to day maintenance problems of life with equilibrium. When we like ourselves, setbacks and disappointments can be overcome. It is easier for us to deal with problems and problem people. It makes us pleasanter to be around, less defensive, and more understanding. It gives us hope and confidence that we can overcome whatever difficulties pass our way.

Self esteem is a treasure we must have and hold if we are to feel the benefits of our full potential.

We all have self esteem. It is how we think of ourselves. We have been around ourselves long enough to develop an opinion about where we rank on the self esteem scale. We know what makes us feel proud and what makes us feel diminished. We can feel confident in some situations and with some people and just the opposite with others. How we feel about ourselves determines how we relate to those around us and influences our demeanor. Will we be assertive or withdrawn? Will we be active or passive? Will we feel happy or sad? Are we in control or being controlled?

Self esteem is the element that makes us feel as though we deserve and receive love and that we are capable of accomplishing good things for ourselves. It is the wonderful feeling that we are worthwhile for no other reason than that we are.

Other words we use reflect our self esteem. We may refer to self worth. What value do we have as an individual? What contribution do we make to the world in which we live? There is self image. This is how we see ourselves. How do we look? How do we feel about our appearance? If we have high self esteem we will feel good about our worth and our image. We may wish for more of the idealized physical beauty, but not having it does not keep us from functioning with purpose and security.

Self esteem begins with our first breath and continues with us for as long as we live. The hope is that as we mature we also become more accepting of ourselves, more appreciative of our skills, and even fond of our foibles, so that our self esteem grows throughout life.

Much of our self esteem as a child develops because of the way we were treated. If we were regarded with love and admiration we will think we were sensational. If we were continually criticized and corrected our self esteem will have suffered.

There comes a time in life when we become responsible for our own self esteem. We own our attitudes, feelings, actions, and choices. We choose how we act. We choose those with whom we associate. We choose our responses. We choose what we learn. Are we developing in a way that enhances our self esteem, or in a way that makes us wonder about ourselves?

It is easier for us if we were nurtured towards self esteem by admiring caretakers. This gives us a head start in life. However, at any age we can receive help or help others with self esteem. We all know adults who once were schoolmates of ours who have completely changed. Remember the class wimp, who on becoming a college president, began acting with assuredness and decision? This person chose to learn skills that increased self esteem. Her self image changed. Her self worth changed. Her self esteem shot up! People treated her differently.

It is much easier to work with elderly residents who have had a lifetime of excellent self esteem that has not wavered as their life style has changed. This is not always a realistic expectation for nursing home residents. In the first place all of us have severe challenges to our self esteem during our life time. Charted on a graph, our self esteem would look like a company displaying business reversals over a course of several years. In the second place, self esteem is often woefully low for persons who have to give up independence and become dependent on strangers. In the third place, some people never have developed good self esteem at any time in their lives.

Our job is defined. We must enhance the self esteem of the nursing home resident. It can be done. It has been done. We will do it.

AREAS OF SELF ESTEEM

Our self esteem is not only based on our perceptions of how we are regarded by others, but on what we have decided is most important to us. I refer here to the basic values we hold dear. We all have certain particulars to which we assign priorities. Values differ widely from person to person, family to family, and culture to culture. We grow up with values. We inherit values. Values shape our lives, our thoughts, our choices, our impressions, and our actions. One person may give the most merit to education or position, another to money or muscles. Values are learned. Values are a matter of interest and attention. Certain values appeal to us, others lack appeal or are even appalling to us. Some cultural values we may adopt are:

Money

Status in our culture often seems to be awarded on the basis of monetary value. How much do we make? How much are we worth? All things being equal, the persons with financial influence are given more respect.

Power

One of the most popular television programs on prime time deals with power. We are not always so concerned about how a person achieved their advantage. We are simply fascinated by their ability to wield it.

Influence

One of our catch phrases is, "It's not what you know, but who you know." We look up to the person who has connections. The "I can get it for you wholesale" mentality is alive and well in our society.

Appearance

We have only to look at the advertisements on television and in popular magazines to know that being thin, young, and having sex appeal are the sure routes to feeling good about ourselves. Take off pounds, dress right, cream away wrinkles, smell good, and people will compete for our company.

Fame

Our heroes are those whose names are in the public eye. We are impressed when we meet someone who has nationwide name recognition, no matter the reason for the fame. We all tend to be name droppers.

Sports

Who are among the most highly paid employees in this country? Sports has its own channel on television and is a major part of many of the other networks' programming. An entire section of the newspaper is devoted to sports. Sports figures make headlines.

Families are influenced by society's values, but often have their own set of values. Some familial values that may weigh in our lives and in our daily decisions are:

Popularity

Most parents want their children to be well liked. They worry if their children don't have friends. They are pleased when they are members of clubs, elected to office, or selected for honors. Overall most people want to be liked and having friends is a tangible symbol that they are.

Education

There is status in higher education. In some households the only way to achieve status is to do well in school and progress to ever higher academic achievement.

Loyalty

Family loyalty is an expected given. However, loyalty can be, and sometimes is, interpreted as meaning that one supports all family members, right or wrong, and that questioning any decision or action or even venturing outside of the family for friends or interests is a sure sign of disloyalty.

Material Things

We all like a nice home, reliable car, some of the latest gadgets, and good looking clothes. Some judge success, quality of life, and acceptability by the number of trendy things a person has. The latest, the best, and the most are the bywords for status in some families.

Health

As important as health is to everyone, some families see that as the ticket to inclusion. Unhealthy people, those with chronic illnesses, physical disabilities or deformities are simply not valued in such families.

Religion

Religion has its stalwart supporters and spirituality is a part of the lives of most people. However, some families can't accept wayward members who do not embrace their particular religious beliefs.

Cleanliness

Cleanliness for some is a doctrine that limits their entire way of life. Some families have cut off visiting members who cannot maintain their proscribed level of cleanliness.

Humanity

Concern for and giving to our fellow human beings is the overriding virtue in some family systems. To stray from this way is seen by some as having false values.

Achievement

How high can we go? In some families that is not high enough. The top person is the only one who has made it. Any job that doesn't provide evidence that the person is getting ahead is not a job worth considering. The contented, salaried person is seen as a loser.

These are some of the many values that influence our lives and our self esteem. What seems important to the people important to us is a basis for how we judge others and ourselves. All of these values will be represented in the nursing home residents. Often we make decisions about another person's worth based on the things that we value. Consequently, if we value athletic ability above all, we will not have high regard for someone who does not possess this attribute. We must realize that values are subjective, personal, and a product of our background and beliefs. We must learn to accept people for their values, not ours.

If we look, we will see values in action in the nursing home.

Ms. A's nursing assistant was in a hurry, couldn't find Ms. A's shoes, and dressed her in a pair of attractive, comfortable slippers. Ms. A was outraged. She knew she had shoes. It was not her custom to go out dressed in bedroom clothes. Wheelchair bound, she could not get down and look for the shoes herself. She was mortified to be seen in what she considered a practically undressed state. She was nasty and unpleasant to everyone she saw, but particularly to her nursing assistant. Ms. A's value was appearance. She could content herself for hours applying her makeup and selecting her jewelry. She wanted to look the way she had looked for ninety years. She was not about to change her value at this late date. Her self esteem was tied up in her looks.

Ms. B was taught that one never went out with wet hair. This was a health rule that she enforced with her own children. It was felt that if one exposed a wet head to the elements one was sure to catch a cold. Ms. B valued the folk medicine she grew up with and believed in it. Whenever she was showered her hair was washed and tied up behind her head and left to air dry. She was then taken to the dining room or the activity room. On days when her hair was wet she was cantankerous, loud, and disturbing to the other residents. She was sure she would get sick because she was doing the very thing she knew would lead to health problems. How much simpler it would have been to honor Ms. B's values and towel or blow dry her hair, or let her stay in her room until it dried.

When residents' values are compromised it is a blow to their self esteem. Both values and self esteem are threatened when a resident enters a nursing home. This is because of major changes in the residents' life such as:

1. Change in life style.
2. Loss of independence.
3. Loss of home.
4. Threat to some values.
5. Physical impairment.
6. Loss of friends and relatives.
7. Physical changes.
8. Health problems.
9. Loss of role.
10. Financial difficulties.

Many residents suffer all of the above. Mr. C is an example.

Mr. C moved from his familiar neighborhood and home where he had raised his family to a condominium to make maintenance and upkeep easier for him. Shortly after the move his wife died from a heart attack. Her pension check stopped. As he was recovering from this loss he suffered a stroke. Medical costs escalated. Since his children worked and could not care for him at home he was placed in a nursing facility. He no longer was able to function independently. This had been his value all his life. He had even had his own business rather than work for someone else. Now he needed help for all his activities of daily living as he was confined to a wheelchair. He had good care, but for the most part was not allowed to make decisions, even those affecting his own daily schedule. His children no longer came to him for advice. They gave him pep talks on how he should adjust to his new life.

Since Mr. C didn't have much left of what made him feel good about himself, he needed a lot of help from everyone to develop new areas of self esteem and to build on important, but neglected qualities he still possessed. He no longer represented the successful, happy, busy, retired man interacting with friends, neighbors, and relatives. He saw himself as a dependent has-been tolerating each day because he had no control over his fate. His picture of himself was drastically altered from his ideal to a nightmare reality. We couldn't call in the marketing people to sell him a new value, but we could help him adjust to what he had that was good and aid him in his enjoyment of those qualities.

We build on strengths. Mr. C still had feelings. He still had a family concerned about him. Whether or not he liked it, he was still alive. Keeping Mr. C in mind, think about what affects our self esteem. Our self esteem is a product of:

1. Our perception of our success or failure.
2. How other people treat us.
3. Our own value system.
4. How we see our role and place in life.
5. Our looks.
6. Our abilities.
7. The respect we feel is due us and whether or not we receive it.
8. Earning capability.
9. Financial status.
10. Where we live.
11. How we live.
12. Who we know.
13. What we own.

14. Our friends.

15. Physical well-being.

16. Feelings of security.

17. How we see ourselves in relation to those around us.

18. Our own feelings about ourselves.

When one of the above is threatened, our self esteem is threatened. I recall a friend who was told by his weekend guest that he would not visit anymore because he was too fussy, too overprotective of his child, and worried too much. He felt terrible. He felt friendless. He figured the relationship was destroyed because of his own failings. He needed something to boost his self esteem. The next day he was talking with other friends, getting reassurance that he was liked, still did have admirers, and that he wasn't as bad as his departing guest had said he was. He carefully went around rebuilding his self esteem.

The elderly will look for reaffirmation too. It may not be as easy for them because when they lose a major portion of self esteem, it is hard to find a place to start rebuilding. We can help them find areas of competence and self admiration in one of the eighteen general areas listed. In all people there is some positive point that we can stress and make important to us and, thus, to them.

Back to Mr. C. There was strength in his family ties. He had a history of good self esteem. He knew how to get along with others. He could be treated with respect and consideration. Mr. C could achieve success as he learned to do all that he could for himself. We could emphasize his worth and his skills and concentrate on his value to his family and the value of developing as many independent skills as possible.

LOW SELF ESTEEM

Having low self esteem is miserable. We feel miserable. We act miserable. We make those around us miserable. Some of the symptoms of low self esteem are:

1. Selfishness.
2. Fear.
3. Protective of self.
4. Insecurity.
5. Anger.
6. Bragging.
7. Jealousy.
8. Possessiveness.
9. Seeking constant approval.
10. Bullying.
11. Prejudice.
12. Easily threatened.
13. Shame.
14. Overly sensitive to criticism.
15. Need to be the boss.
16. Nonassertive.
17. Pretentious.
18. Anxious.
19. Blaming.
20. Conceited.
21. Dependent.

22. Suffering fatigue and other physical symptoms.

23. Self consciousness.

24. Cynicism.

Selfishness

When we feel insecure and needy we hold on to what we have with tenacity. We fear that if we let anything go we will be further diminished. We cannot give material things, unqualified love, admiration, or assistance without thinking, "What's in it for me?"

Fear

When we suffer low self esteem we feel we are not in control. Consequently, we fear that anything bad that can happen, can happen to us — and probably will. We fear not only for ourselves and our families, but our fears can encompass everything and everybody. This concern for the world may appear as compassion. Instead it is an all embracing fear and expectation of doom.

Protective of Self

High self esteem does not mean that we take foolhardy chances. It does mean that we take some risk. We have to risk ourselves and our perceived security in order to grow, progress, and learn. Persons with low self esteem will protect themselves in every venture, be it physical, emotional, or material.

Insecurity

If we have overwhelming fears we are always insecure. If we are insecure we feel we are at the mercy of others, of the unknown, of fate.

Anger

If anything can harm us and we have no defense against those forces we feel frustrated and angry. Our anger, if we have low self esteem, is often expressed inappropriately, uncontrollably, and is misdirected. It can be exhibited by lack of cooperation, sarcasm, insults, resistance, passivity, and physical and verbal striking out.

Bragging

When we have low self esteem we don't believe anyone really notices our value or notes our successes. Actually, we aren't sure our achievements are worthwhile. Thus, we must brag to convince others of our ability, but most of all to convince ourselves.

Jealousy

If we had what other people have we think we would have great self esteem. If they had nothing we would have more than they and we would be better than they are. Too bad this is such an apparent fallacy.

Possessiveness

We don't want to share people, things, or ideas. If we give up anything it lessens us and our self esteem suffers. If people involved with us, (they don't necessarily have to be intimates) show independent actions or interests in others it feels like rejection to us.

Seeking Constant Approval

When we don't feel good about ourselves we can't risk allowing others to have negative feelings about us. Without approval from others we get depressed and can reach the point of being nonfunctional. The need for approval can become so extreme that the slightest frown or indication of disapproval will induce despair and self abrogation.

Bullying

If we can push others around it must mean that we are potent people. Bullying is like a drug. Once the effect wears off we have to bully again to keep our self esteem intact.

Prejudice

Prejudice is made for people with low self esteem. If a group of people can be considered faulty the people who feel uncertain about their own place in the scheme of things can feel better about themselves. By looking down on a selected few, laughing at their ineptness, or seeing them as undesirable, the persons with low self esteem can take false pride in being members of a more successful group.

Easily Threatened

Remember idling behind drivers at an intersection and waiting for them to pull out into the traffic so we can complete our turn? The people who can't make the decision to drive on when the road looks clear symbolizes those with low self esteem. Those people are so easily thwarted that a car on the horizon seems a threat. They are threatened by two people walking and talking together. They see conspiracies and plots all around. A quiet "no" may seem a declaration of war to them.

Shame

People with low self esteem are ashamed to share family or personal background because they think such tidbits of information may be embarrassing. Someone may poke fun at them. They do not dare to express an opinion as they may be laughed at. Common human functions and frailties are a source of self flagellation for them.

Overly Sensitive to Criticism

Most of us exhibit only mild chagrin when we are told of a minor mistake such as being in the wrong place at the wrong time or giving slightly inaccurate information. It is annoying and can be inconvenient, but having these errors pointed out is no major denunciation to our self esteem. Those lacking in self esteem will see this as a failing that reconfirms their total inability to get anything right.

Need to be the Boss

One way we can compensate for low self esteem is to have power. This does not necessarily raise our self esteem, but can give us the appearance of being held in esteem. When people always need to be in charge, consider their need to have others build them up. This is not the same as the person who is able to lead because of ability and knowledge.

Nonassertive

The doormat types can't feel very good about themselves if they let everyone walk on them, can they? Nevertheless, it is one way to get attention as almost everyone passes their way.

Pretentious

If we pretend we're better than others maybe we will be. At least this is the hope of the person with low self esteem.

Anxious

When we are under stress certain physiological changes take place in our body. Our adrenalin flows. Our heart beats faster. We may feel tremors. We get tense. We are anxious. When we have low self esteem we are unsure and uncomfortable in most situations. Anxiety occurs. The physical and emotional toll goes on and on.

Blaming

If it's someone else's fault I am in the clear. And if my self esteem is low, it is too much of a risk to take the blame. Others might disapprove of me and that I could not bear.

Conceited

What appears to be conceit and total self centeredness is a defensive mechanism for people with low self esteem. Who will acknowledge them, they think. They feel responsible for their own self aggrandizement.

Dependent

Since I can't take care of myself, you must do it for me. Self esteem is so low, dependent people need others to make them feel like a whole person.

Suffering Fatigue and other Physical Complaints

Low self esteem makes us uncertain. This uncertainty causes stress. The constant stress makes our body work harder. Fatigue develops. Other physical complaints such as breathing problems, dizziness, stomach and backaches, and heart irregularities are common. Besides it is easier for us to focus on tangible physical complaints than deal with ourselves, our feelings, and our relationships.

Self Consciousness

It seems incongruous that someone who has low self esteem imagines that everyone notices what they do, but such is the case. Of course, they also exaggerate all their own responses, see them as awkward, get more self conscious, and become more awkward.

Cynicism

Everybody and everything is rotten and always will be is the theme of the cynical person. If there is the possibility that someone will act in their own interest or that an event will go wrong, you can be sure that the cynic will predict the worst.

This evidence of poor self esteem runs the gamut of human emotions. Most are not uncommon in any of us. Some are even appropriate at times. But when one lives, day to day, with any of the basically negative attitudes that cause behavior problems, unhappy relationships develop. These nonproductive alliances usually confirm the residents' feelings of low self esteem and perpetuates the difficult behavior.

For example:

Mr. D complained about every person in the facility. Some were too loud, others were out of it. He would insult them to their faces. The nursing assistants and nurses were too rough, too slow, or too dumb. All the activities were geared to idiots. By putting everyone and everything down he tried to point out that he was better. That was his way of trying to make himself feel good. Obviously it didn't work. The staff avoided him when possible and the residents were frightened of him.

Ms. E did not care how she looked. She refused to go to the beauty parlor. She would not get dressed. Her attitude was one of hopelessness. She saw no reason to look her best. She felt no one cared and she did not care either.

Ms. F spent the day smiling and telling everyone how pretty they were and how wonderful they were to her. She tried to pay the nursing home staff and encouraged other residents to eat her goodies. She always wanted to help out. Her constant praise became an irritant as it was so injudicious. She was in the way when she ineptly attempted to assist other residents. Her efforts to ingratiate herself only made her annoying.

Mr. G followed every introduction with the statement that he had made and lost a million dollars, and made it again. This preceded his recital of all the famous people he knew and historical events he witnessed. His fellow residents were quite outspoken about their feelings regarding his braggadocio.

Ms. H never said hello. She always said, "My hands are cold." She never said goodbye. Instead it was, "I have to lie down because of my back." Soon her many physical complaints were ignored. Everyone had heard them and had learned that they could not be remedied.

Ms. I could not leave her room. She could not be away from her bathroom. Her daughter might visit. Her doctor was coming. She needed to watch a television program. When forced into the hallway her fear was apparent. Staff finally stopped asking her to go places.

All of these are symptoms of low self esteem. Residents were demonstrating that they did not have high regard for themselves nor a constructive way of managing their feelings. The end result of their behavior only reinforced their fears that they were not worthy of respect and esteem. Since they did not have other coping mechanisms to solve this problem for themselves they continued to rely on their old patterns, trying harder and harder to achieve that which was beyond their reach. As they intensified their behavior, they received more negative feedback. The old reliable vicious circle was doing fine. About all we can say is that it was a familiar way for the residents and they were accustomed to the reactions.

We'd like to break into this pattern and assist the residents in getting out of these unhappy situations. We can do this by responding to positive aspects of their behavior or personalities and ignoring the unpleasant way in which they conduct themselves.

HIGH SELF ESTEEM

High self esteem means that we have a healthy sense of self respect and caring. It is an energizing form of self love that does not involve egotism. It is a self satisfaction that does not mean that our way is the only way. People with high self esteem usually exhibit the following qualities.

1. Self control.
2. Ability to share.

3. Feelings of competence.
4. Ability to ask for help.
5. Ability to make decisions.
6. Appreciation of own worth.
7. Respect for others.
8. Hopefulness.
9. Can trust others and are trustworthy.
10. Accepts own and others' feelings.
11. Can accept and give compliments.
12. Interest in others.
13. Accept others for what they are.
14. Feel they can influence what happens in their lives.
15. Can listen to others.

Self Control

We may feel like punching someone but we can control this impulse by considering the context. We can think about the other person's real intent, not taking everything personally, weighing the consequences, and selecting the appropriate behavior for the circumstances.

Ability to Share

We can share our belongings, but more importantly, we are secure enough to share our thoughts, feelings, and follies.

Feelings of Competence

We know we aren't great at everything and not even good at many things. We do know that we do well in some areas and can get by in others. We are willing to try what seems interesting if our self esteem is OK.

Ability to Ask for Help

When help is needed we can go to the appropriate provider. We don't feel that they will look down on us, reject us, or take advantage of our vulnerability. If possible, we are pleased to help in return.

Ability to Make Decisions

When we feel good about ourselves we know we can make decisions we can live with. Consequently, we can decide, act on our decisions, and never look back.

Appreciation of Own Worth

It is nice to have others appreciate us and tell us so. Still, if we have high self esteem we can know we have a valuable place in life without having to have others continually remind us of this fact.

Respect for Others

Like charity, respect begins at home. When we respect ourselves we can respect others.

Hopefulness

Hope is not just blind faith that everything will turn out all right, but a belief that life will continue to be interesting, people will be generally supportive, and we will be able to cope.

Can Trust Others and are Trustworthy

If we have to guard ourselves continually and in all areas, life becomes a very bristly and an uncomfortable affair. If we can let ourselves trust judiciously we can relax and enjoy. By the same token, if we have confidence that we will do as we say, can fulfill our obligations, and that others can count on us, we have high self esteem.

Accepts Own and Others' Feelings

We can recognize that all healthy people have a range of normal feelings. Our feelings are not good or bad, just real and human. We accept these qualities in ourselves and in others and feel good about them.

Can Accept and Give Compliments

When someone tells us something nice about ourselves or our possessions we don't look for ulterior motives, become embarrassed by the focus of the attention, or feign modesty. We are delighted with what we do or say, how we look, or when what we own pleases others. Conversely we want to let others know when they bring us happiness or capture our admiration.

Interest in Others

When we feel content with ourselves our world expands. We don't need to keep our attention within narrow bounds. We can increase our interests to include others and through them, learn and grow. We can show concern, compassion, and pleasure for others.

Accept Others for What They Are

If we accept ourselves, we can accept others. We don't have to make them over to meet our preconceived design of what they should be. An individuals' uniqueness is prized.

Feel They Can Influence What Happens in Their Lives

No sense of hopelessness here. Feelings of self worth give us a feeling of control. We deserve and expect consideration and respect. We can exert ourselves without overpowering. We are responsible for much of what happens to us.

Can Listen to Others

Ever tried to talk to people who only let us finish a sentence so they can tell us what happened to them? Those with high self esteem do not have the need to dominate a conversation. They can listen to others because:

a. They are interested in others.

b. They recognize the need for others to express themselves.

c. They realize they can learn from others.

d. They want to help.

e. They are secure enough that they don't need to dominate every conversation.

Mr. J was unable to walk. He used a wheelchair to get around. He was barely able to swallow. He drooled. His voice was just a whisper. Nonetheless, everyone in the nursing home knew and greeted him. He attended events, visited other residents, asked riddles, kept abreast with current events, got along well with his roommate, and had a good sense of humor. He was an asset in any situation.

Mr. K had severe and unsightly cancer growths that caused his face to be grotesque. He communicated with a magic slate. But no one ever questioned his ability. He was alert, involved, and included. His compassion, concern, and pleasant personality came through by way of his eyes, his body language, and his manner. When he succumbed to his illness he was truly mourned.

When we have high self esteem we assign value to our and other peoples' lives.

Chapter II

ENHANCING SELF ESTEEM

ATMOSPHERE

Emotional Setting

We are all intimately familiar with the struggle for self esteem. Most of us look for it all of our lives. We find it sometimes in some places with some people and often within ourselves. We know what makes us feel good and what makes us feel at the bottom of the heap. Because we have this daily acquaintance with self esteem none of what is written here is actually unknown to us. Mainly we will be conceptualizing what we know and applying it to the nursing home residents.

To create an atmosphere that enhances the residents' self esteem we must first take care of our own feelings. I had a supervisor who told me that if I wasn't feeling good about myself and others (I was in the people pleasing business) I should stay home from work. This sounded great to me! However, I soon determined that I was going to have to tackle the feeling good issue from a different direction than missing work. Her message was clear. If I couldn't do the job, I shouldn't report for it. If I didn't report for it, I wouldn't have the job. I had to accomplish the task of feeling good about myself so that I could feel good about others and at the same time keep my job. My attitude and mood set the tone for interactions that took place around me. I controlled the atmosphere in that way. Because I could create a positive atmosphere, I got more positive responses from other people. I did learn that everyone does not respond to the positive approach. I was not the only factor in their lives. They had other events and contacts during the day or during their lives that made them react negatively no matter what I did. I learned that they were doing what they were doing for themselves and not to me. When I sorted this out I stopped taking their moods and behaviors personally. Their negative feelings did not disrupt my self esteem. Since their problems did not effect me personally, I did not have to let them upset me. I did not have to pass these feelings on to the next person. I did not have to take it out on an innocent party.

Attitudes can be very contagious. If someone has a bad attitude they are perfectly willing to share it. If I let it rub off on me I infect the next person or persons with whom I deal. In this way a negative atmosphere quickly corrupts the surroundings. This is particularly dangerous in a closed environment such as a nursing home. The residents are most susceptible to the attitude and atmosphere around them. We can make it a positive one. We can make the crucial difference. We can leave our self esteem problems at home and concentrate on developing an atmosphere that makes those around us feel good. In this way we can influence those we work with in a pleasant and powerful way. This spirals. Our enjoyment and appreciation will be disseminated to others.

Acknowledge that we have worth. Acknowledge that everyone has worth. Not one of us is without merit from the day we are born until the day we die. No matter what we do, we are all of value. We are worthwhile when we are helpless, sick, young, old, or asleep, just as we are worthwhile when we are active, employed, and carrying out responsibilities. This worth is always with all of us. It never changes. It never goes away.

We cannot feel our own worth to any effective extent or even lead an emotionally healthy life without positive strokes. Positive strokes do not have to involve elaborate compliments or physical intimacy. A positive stroke can mean an approving smile, a knowing glance, an acknowledging wave, or a pat on the shoulder. Some good strokes for our fellow workers and the nursing home residents are careful listening, hugs, compliments, and encouragement.

The best stroke of all is to have our dignity and pride respected and our opinions considered. The nursing home residents want and need this just as we all do. Without it they lose their pride and the symptoms of poor self esteem are exhibited.

Physical Setting

Not all nursing homes can be new and modern. All can be clean and cheerful. It is unfortunate, but most facility applicants feel as though they are being relegated to an undesirable setting when they must live in a nursing home. Consequently, it is important to give the residents the message that they are living in a terrific place. Help them achieve pride in their surroundings. The unspoken message should be that the facility is a great place to live. I once heard a talk given by a nursing home administrator in which she described the amenities and the opportunities offered in her place of work. She made it sound like a resort hotel. All of us in the room could hardly wait to visit, and if we hadn't known she was talking about a nursing home, would have made reservations and given her a deposit.

This doesn't mean that we have to assault people with the hard sell and force them to comply with the party line that everything is wonderful. It does mean that the advantages of being where food, entertainment, and loving care are provided are made evident. If the staff can represent the facility as a good place to work, if they are proud to be associated with it, and if they can see the benefits, they can help the residents develop similar attitudes. They can brag about the skill, background, education, dedication, and number of staff members. They can point out the beauty of the grounds, the building, the decorations, or the furniture. They can share their enjoyment of the food, the activities, the recreational opportunities, or the length of the waiting list. It makes us feel better about ourselves if we think we are smart enough to live in a place others also want to be. Association with success makes us feel successful too. If the physical atmosphere gives the impression of something desirable, elegant, and special, people will think we are lucky to work or stay in such an enviable environment. If our surroundings are marvelous, we must be marvelous too!

Sometimes our self esteem is tied up in our possessions or the things that have value to us because they elicit important memories. An atmosphere of respect is due belongings because acquisitions often represent a part of the residents. The residents should feel that their items of personal memorabilia are valued, that their property is safe, can be used by them, and kept near them. Personal property can enhance residents' self esteem if they are allowed to cherish it and staff members recognize its worth and meaning to the residents.

Mr. L's family never visited him. The one strong relationship he had in the nursing home was his girlfriend. Then she died. He was so hurt he refused to get involved with anyone else. He gave every indication that he had no reason to live. His one sparkle of interest came when a church group gave him a wreath for his door. This he loved. He showed it to everyone. He was animated. He smiled. He returned to his sulking despondency when nursing home rules precluded him from putting it on his door with a nail (understandable). No one suggested any other way to display it. He was too defeated to think of an alternative way. Thus we see that Mr. L's self esteem was increased when someone found him valuable enough to be the recipient of a gift. It was further enhanced when he could show it to others and receive their attention and admiration for his possession. It was dashed when his plans for his new belonging could not be carried out.

Ms. M had beautiful lounging clothes. Her sister always made sure that she was dressed in lovely attire. She was not a pleasant woman, but always got attention because her appearance was so attractive. This helped her with her self esteem. More and more she responded to the admiration of others and soon was carrying herself with obvious pride.

Relationships

Our associations contribute to our self esteem. If we remember back to high school we recall how we all envied the "in" group. None of us wanted to be nerds. Recollect how our parents concerned themselves about our friends. They wanted them to be above reproach as they knew that our friends influenced us and that we were judged by our associations. Such has it always been in life. We still are judged by the company we keep. We still like to be with people we admire and respect and who are compatible with us. We don't want to be ashamed of our friends or have them ashamed of us. So it is in a nursing home. It is not always possible to let the residents select their own roommates, but they should be situated so that they are not with roommates who shatter their self esteem.

Ms. N shared a room with a woman who was incontinent. Although Ms. N understood that her roommate could not help this, she felt that she too was considered to be unable and dependent because she was put in a room with a person who needed such help. She was afraid to express her concerns as she did not want them verified. Her self esteem seemed to dissipate only to bounce back when she was given another roommate. At that time she said with relief that she worried that she was thought to be failing fast and that was why she had been placed with the previous roommate. Her next roommate was capable. So Ms. N thought she too must be an able person and functioned like one.

Mr. O would never invite anyone to his room because his roommate was disoriented and yelled inappropriately.

For reasons known only to Mr. O he took his roommate's infirmities as a reflection on him such as a child with an alcoholic parent is embarrassed to invite other children to her home.

Ms. P had a roommate who criticized her constantly. She was too noisy, too slow, and stupid. Although the staff tried to help Ms. P ignore the abusive roommate, she could not. She took all the insults to heart and her self esteem plummeted.

Ms. Q and her roommate liked each other until they tried to live together. They found that they had altogether different habit patterns. One slept late. The other liked to watch television in the morning. One had a lot of company. The other cherished her privacy. They tolerated each other with some forbearance for awhile, and then became argumentative and insulting. Ms. Q felt she was a failure because she could not succeed with her chosen roommate. Her self esteem suffered.

On the other hand, roommates can help self esteem if together they form a bond of mutual trust and admiration, if they support each other, and if a relationship develops that gives them a feeling of security. They end up feeling good about themselves and each other.

In an atmosphere where relationships are allowed to develop and flourish, self esteem can grow. Residents can become attached to their roommates and choose and make friends.

Ms. R and Mr. S are an example of a close friendship. When they attended the oral autobiography class given at the nursing home they were asked to tell about the best time of their life. They both said it was the present time for them. When asked why they giddily explained it was because they had found each other.

STAFF MEMBERS' ATTITUDES AND BEHAVIORS

Staff Self Esteem

The tone of any encounter is set by the staff member. Worries regarding family, career, and social contacts work away at us, erode our psyche, and have no place in our relationship with people we are paid to help. Getting outside ourselves and allowing ourselves to be distracted is a healing exercise. Being able to help others helps us with our own self esteem. We should be able to get self satisfaction from our job and feel the pleasure of being able to give to others in a situation where our giving makes the difference.

Our own giving and concern for others is our opportunity to model behavior for those in our care. The nursing home residents must identify with the nursing home staff for lack of other role models. If they see the people they depend upon being grumpy, self centered, negative, and mean, they may well decide that this is the behavior and attitude that is expected in the environment. We can be what we would like them to be. If anyone asks us why we are always cheerful and willing we can tell them that we are setting an example. We can say that we are acting the way we wish everyone would act. Our self control and role modeling will enhance our own self esteem and increase our feelings of competence.

So let's go all the way. Let's continue our model behavior by always being polite and courteous, thinking of the needs of the residents. This does not mean that we should put our own needs completely aside, or that we should make unreasonable demands on ourselves. It means that we treat those in our care with kindness and concern and we always remember the social amenities such as:

1. Saying please and thank you when making any requests and achieving compliance.

2. Respecting privacy and not intruding without asking or explaining why it is necessary.

3. Observing individual preferences and personal time frames as much as possible.

4. Apologizing for inconveniences.

5. Admitting mistakes.

Etiquette, which means proper and accepted behavior, helps the recipients' self esteem as it makes them feel as though they are worthy of our esteem and consideration. They feel as though we consider them deserving of respectful deportment and will look on themselves as people who should behave in an appropriate way.

Negatives to Positives

We have more than enough aggravation in our lives. We are all pretty good at dwelling on them. One thing most of us should have learned by now is that focusing on that which irritates us only makes it larger than life. Constantly bringing the unwanted behavior or attitude to another's attention only reinforces the problem and increases the incidence of the unwanted behavior. We should also have learned that it is not easy to change another person. Any of us who have tried to change our relatives or friends to meet our standards know that it is a totally thankless and unrewarding job.

So, how do we change the negatives to positives? We focus on ourselves. We change our way of thinking and/or behaving.

Ms. T was the most irritating person. She never smiled. When she was through drinking, she threw her glass on the floor. She stopped her wheelchair in the middle of the hallway, effectively blocking everyone's way. She always asked, "When do we eat?" The residents and staff tried to avoid her, but she always seemed to be in the way or asking for something. The most common comment regarding this resident was, "Oh, her again." One day she went, uninvited, to an activity that included trivia questions. To everyone's amazement she participated and exhibited good knowledge of trivia names and dates. At first her answers were sullen, but as she began to get recognition for her ability she became more animated. Since this was such a singular event, news of her success traveled quickly. Soon she was receiving compliments and comments on what she had done. Everyone had found a new and positive side to Ms. T's personality. Her irritating behavior continued, but it didn't bother everybody as much as they now saw her as a person with more facets to her being. There were aspects of her that could be admired. She became interesting. As staff and residents concentrated on her positive performance, she showed this side more often. The negatives were not so frequently in evidence.

If we identify and praise the positive parts of the residents' personalities, they will begin to respond to our reinforcers and develop these characteristics further. To the residents' detriment, we often call attention to the negative behaviors and attitudes and reinforce them instead. Even if there is no change in the recipients of our praise, it helps us to cope if we can find something in the residents that we like. It makes it easier for us to care for and about the residents when we acknowledge to ourselves and to the resident that we have found something to appreciate. The benefit of this approach is that we treat the persons better and they grow in self esteem. This growth may start from a small seed, such as a superficial compliment on the color of their eyes. We are susceptible to admiration, even if it is admiration of something over which we have no control. Nonetheless, it feels good and none of us get enough of it.

Never see people or situations as hopeless or beyond endurance. Try to find the good that can come from the situation. Totally bedridden, dependent people have life itself to live for. They may have their memories. They may enjoy the touch of their attendants. They may like the pattern the sun makes on the wall. They may enjoy the sound of a bird singing, or people walking down the hallway. Pity does not convey esteem. Realize that life is life and while there is breath these people are making a contribution to life. This is giving proper esteem.

Nursing home work seems to train us to zero in on problems. All our paper work is geared to the negative. Charts contain problem lists. Our care plans start out by stating the problem and then go on to say how WE will solve it. The progress notes deal primarily with what went wrong and what has to be done for the resident. Special consultation and attention are required only when all is not well. We look for the weaknesses and work at compensating for them. None of this is wrong. We need to know where we can help and have a direction for doing so. But when all our attention is given to what has gone awry, we neglect what is going right. The good and the healthy are allowed to fade because we don't have time to help these parts to flourish. We think that the functioning aspects can prosper without us. This may not be so. What is neglected can atrophy as does a muscle that is not used. Use it or lose it!

Why don't we have strength lists in the charts? This is a list of what the residents do well. This is what should be encouraged. We can build on the positives of the residents. Let's note what we appreciate in the residents. How about an esteem list? We can write down what the residents like about themselves so that we can help them keep that measure of self esteem. We can pinpoint areas where we can help them build up their self esteem. Often we are most successful in boosting others' self esteem by starting the process on the basis of what they already like about themselves. It is easier to build on positives than try to get rid of the negatives and then start from scratch. From scratch may be the way to bake a good cake, but it is not the best way to develop personal good feelings.

In every way possible, look for the positives. Emphasize strengths.

Ms. U was labeled a tattle tale by the staff and other residents. She apparently felt it her responsibility to let the staff know when residents were where they should not be or were doing something she suspected was unacceptable. She also tended to remind the staff of their duties. Her unwanted, but correct information, was never welcomed by anyone. This made her more persistent in telling as she was determined that her admonitions be heard. During one care plan meeting Ms. U's habit of interfering was discussed as a problem to be solved. A new nurse mentioned that she found Ms. U's observations helpful, accepted them as stated, and although she didn't base her treatments on them, told her thank you. Ms. U did not nag at her. The new employee found Ms. U's reminder a nice check as she was learning her new duties. The nurse accepted Ms. U's reports as those of a concerned party and treated them accordingly. Since the old approach of trying to get Ms. U to bug off was not working, the staff decided to try the method of giving Ms. U credit for her contributions to the running of an orderly community. As it turned out, Ms. U was delighted that the staff was finally listening to her. She no longer felt the compelling need to nag, follow up or become insistent. Since she felt trusted and included she accepted explanations regarding exceptions in the routines and rules and was satisfied to limit herself to pertinent observations. Her self esteem went up as she got to be a member of the team. This is what she wanted all along. She wanted to promote the well being of the community. She was accustomed to being responsible for her fellow humans. She did not want to lose this role in her life. By switching their attitudes the staff members were able to make what appeared to be a negative habit into a positive action.

Giving Approval Through Identification

You've heard the saying, "Love me, love my dog." My husband is that way about his cat. If someone criticizes this animal (an elderly, bad tempered, ordinary looking alley cat) he takes it personally. Whether or not he should take a personal affront is another issue. The point here is that we do identify with the persons, pets, and possessions in our lives. We bask in reflected glory. If our children receive approbation, we are filled with pride and acknowledge the sensitivity and good judgment of the person who gave the tribute.

The elderly nursing home residents often have few persons and possessions left. That we can find what they have pleasing, pleases them. They will take it as a personal plaudit. They will get a good feeling about themselves. We should be able to find something in relatives and friends that is laudatory. Even the worst of us aren't without some redeeming feature.

Living in a nursing home, depending on the care of strangers, is not what any of us wish for ourselves. As much as we like to consider ourselves unique, we also like to think of ourselves as being a part of human events. Being in a nursing home, in some instances, makes us feel removed from the main stream and held safely away from the normal flow of life. For this reason ordinary likes and dislikes, needs, preferences, and wants become more important. It is the ordinary that attracts us when we are divested of our normal life style. When we have been away from home for a few weeks, even on a pleasant journey, we remember that we were glad to return to our familiar routine, life style, and comforts.

The nursing home residents do a magnificent job of adapting to an entirely new routine and schedule, but the familiar and recognition of what they like has real meaning to them. It is acknowledgment of their personhood.

Mr. V was a recent arrival at the nursing home. He was very cranky in the morning. Most of the staff just tried to stay away until the bad temper wore off. One morning the social worker had to get some information that couldn't wait. Mr. V did not try to be congenial. In a desperate try, she said, "I'm always a bear in the morning too, until I have my coffee." Mr. V actually smiled. He agreed. A cup of coffee first thing in the morning was always the beginning of his day. He hated having everything upset, and missing that amenity started his day with bitterness. The social worker got each of them coffee and their interview went well. From then on he had coffee every morning. His mornings were fine. He made a special tie with the social worker because she too liked coffee, and for the same reason he did. He was thrilled to find someone else with his same predilection. It helped his self esteem to know that he was not alone.

We even like others to recognize and identify with our habits. Many of us have felt emotional relief and acceptance when we have found someone who has had the reactions we have had, who has the same preferences, or even similar experiences. We like to talk with people who have had babies, gotten married, experienced death in the family, fallen in love, or been through some of the same traumatic and joyful events as we have. It gives us someone with whom we can identify and confirmation that our reactions and feelings are within the normal range of human response. It helps us accept ourselves and our feelings. The same goes for our preferences. We enjoy a good conversation with people who like the same kind of music, movies, fashions, or food we choose. If other people like it, it confirms that we are OK. It is as though they are approving of us by having the same taste.

Do Nots

There are some circumstances that threaten our self esteem. Other people can do or say something unintentionally, or on purpose, that totally ruins us. These sort of actions happen throughout our lives and also occur in nursing homes. Consequently, there are some things we simply should not do or say when we are devoting ourselves to the care of nursing home residents. Some of these do nots are:

1. Do not imitate the residents' manner, speech habits, or behavior.
2. Do not threaten.
3. Do not say "I'll be right back," or "Just a minute."
4. Do not compare.
5. Do not set up impossibly competitive situations.
6. Do not get defensive.
7. Do not ignore residents.
8. Do not treat residents as though they were inanimate objects.
9. Do not use sarcasm.
10. Do not be too rigid.
11. Do not criticize.
12. Do not neglect.
13. Do not over-indulge.

Do not imitate the residents' manner, speech habits, or behavior.

Imitation is not always the sincerest form of flattery. It often seems as though someone is poking fun. When residents are repetitive in speech or behavior it is easy to pick up on this and repeat the phrase or act out physical gestures. Don't do it. It is insulting to the residents and the residents' family and friends. Even if the residents do not appear to be aware that this is occurring, they get the feel of the atmosphere and know that something is happening that is not respectful to them. Other residents see and hear that one of them is being treated in an uncaring way. Even though they may laugh and have the same tendency to mimicry they will have an inner concern that if others are treated rudely they may be too. Self esteem cannot grow in such an environment.

Do not threaten.

It is easy to say, "If you don't shape up, I will punish you." We address children that way. It isn't necessarily right for them. It certainly is a wrong way to speak to adults. We don't respond well to threats. The natural way to react is to get defensive, get more stubborn and set in our ways, to justify why we are doing it, or to blame the accuser for making the situation happen.

When Ms. W was told she should never go into anyone's room without permission or she would be restricted to the dining room she immediately denied that she ever did such a thing. Now there was no way to find out if she was looking for something, was lost, or was trying to steal from the other residents. She got defensive and would not budge from her position.

Ms. X smoked in her room. This was not allowed. The nurse said she was to stop or have all her cigarettes removed from her possession. She heard those as fighting words and looked for no solution to the problem other than hiding cigarettes and approaching visitors for handouts.

Mr. Y liked the women and they liked him. That didn't make it appropriate for him to hug and kiss them in public places. It was explained that if he didn't stop this behavior in the activity and sitting rooms he would be expelled from the nursing home. He said it wasn't his fault. The women enticed him and grabbed at him. He was complying to make them happy. He did not make a change in behavior. He made excuses.

Mr. Z was losing weight. If he didn't eat his food the doctor would be called and he would be force fed. Mr. Z said it wasn't his fault he didn't eat. The food was bad. They brought it to him cold. The other residents' eating habits ruined his appetite. It was everyone's fault but his.

All these situations are common in nursing homes. The threatened consequences are realistic. A problem with threats is that once one is made it has to be carried out or the person making the threat loses all credibility. Another difficulty in making a threat is that a threat interferes with problem solving. All of the residents described had problems that caused dilemmas for them and for the nursing home staff. They were not given a chance to approach their problems in a way that might bring them to a point of voluntarily altering their behaviors or creatively clearing up their quandaries. Instead they were put in the position of maintaining their stance that their behavior was the desired and acceptable way to be. It would have been better to confront them with the problem and mutually work for a satisfactory answer.

When we threaten we make the problem ours and take sole responsibility for determining the outcome. Let the problem stay with the perpetrators. Let them struggle with an acceptable solution and work at controlling their behavior.

Mr. AA refused his medicine. His nurse explained why his medicine was prescribed and why it was the staff's responsibility to see that he took it. He was sure that the medicine would make him weak. He had seen his wife deteriorate after she took prescribed medications. Both the nurse and the doctor interpreted the differences between his and his wife's health problems. He agreed that his prescription was probably necessary and complied with the orders. He did not have to get stubborn. The nurse was not forced to be arbitrary. There were no threats. The problem was solved by exploration and agreement.

Do not say "I'll be right back," or "Just a minute."

If we want to make people lose esteem we treat them as though they were last on our list, lie to them, or forget about them. The commonly used phrases "I'll be right back," and "Just a minute," sound like brush offs. When we don't return right away or in a minute (no one ever does) they become lies. When we get occupied with other pressing duties and don't get back to the residents they know they have been forgotten. Since these phrases do nothing but make people upset and angry we should banish them from our vocabulary. Instead we can say specifically what we have to do and when we can get back, giving a realistic time frame. This makes us trustworthy and the residents will feel as though we are treating them as adults instead of as annoyances.

4. *Do not compare.*

My mother always told me that she wished I could close doors as quietly as my childhood friend did. She meant this constructively. It did not mean that she liked my friend better than she liked me. Even so, it felt as though she did.

Residents who are told that they should go to the beauty parlor because their friends do and they look good, end up thinking their friends have more status with us than they do.

If the roommate always says please, or gets up early, or is more cheerful, that's fine. Residents don't want to be told that they should be the same as a favored person. If they wanted to be that way, they could be, as they can see the benefits that go to the roommate because of the behavior.

Do not compare. We may make nice statements about another person, but we don't use that person as an example. If we do, the residents we talk with will think they are being criticized. They will know they've been told that they aren't good enough.

Do not set up impossibly competitive situations.

There is nothing wrong with competition unless it hurts the residents' self esteem. Voluntary competition in games and sports adds interest to life and enhances the self esteem of the winner. This is normal in our culture. Everyone enjoys it. Winning is exhilarating.

The competitive situations I refer to are those where the standards are so high that the residents cannot compete or they end up trying to compete in an area where they cannot succeed.

We set our own high standards when we experience jealousy of Ms. America or Ms. Universe. We may have wished that we could be a rich industrialist or feel a failure because we are not. If our self esteem is damaged by the overwhelming achievements of others, we are setting ourselves up for failure. None of us can achieve all things. The range of competition is too wide. With these feelings we can only falter as our expectations are too great. We cannot compete in every arena. We cannot be what everyone can be. Our competitive urges have to be channeled.

The residents may be able to compete in bowling and volley ball among themselves, but they cannot compete with an olympic sports figure. That fact does not lessen their victory.

Residents may need help in setting competitive limits. Because they can no longer remember all the chess plays does not mean that their self esteem should shatter. They may continue to be good at other games and should be encouraged to enjoy whatever skill they have.

Do not get defensive.

Defensive means that we have a need to protect ourselves. We try to repel an attack. There will be situations where we will be blamed, accused, badgered, or insulted. Such are the vagaries of human interaction. This is particularly rife in a nursing home setting as others are dependent on our care and often unhappy about their dependency. If we want to see a tolerable situation deteriorate, we need only get defensive. What may have been managed becomes impossible.

Instead of getting defensive we can be matter of fact in tone of voice, manner, and body language. We can thwart the attack and not give the residents further reason for offensive action. We can continue to be conversational, caring, and involved. This gives the residents a chance to calm down, to see themselves as persons who can have some control, and to save face. It helps them with their self esteem. Defensive behavior by us threatens their self esteem.

Ms. BB complained that her sheets were dirty and insisted she be brought a clean set. The employee in charge of linens became furious and defended the thoroughness of the laundry operation, declaring that it was impossible for anything to leave there in any but a pristine state. Ms. BB became angry in return and was heard going down the hallway voicing her complaints to all the residents she met and reciting the evidence behind her accusation. The staff member and the resident were both defensive. Trust was lost. Self esteem was hurt.

Mr. CC denounced the Activity Director for not inviting him to any event. Instead of defensively pointing out that this wasn't true she accepted his statement and invited him to attend an activity that same day. The encounter did not end up with each participant feeling insulted, but resulted in a constructive action that made Mr. BB feel as though he had accomplished something.

Do not ignore residents.

Most of us would protest if accused of ignoring those in our care. In fact, we do. Sometimes it is too difficult to hear a soft voice or a garbled vocabulary so we pretend we understand and rush on with our job. Oftentimes we have heard the anxious question so many times we forget that reassurance is necessary each time. The query just doesn't register. Then we are busy and can't be bothered by what appears inconsequential. All of these actions contribute to poor self esteem.

Mr. DD wanted to know the way to the dining room. He asked every day. Staff finally didn't hear his question anymore, made snide remarks such as, "Same place as yesterday," or just took him there without comment. Each time Mr. DD seemed to become more confused and dependent. His dismay with himself appeared to increase. His confidence lessened along with his self esteem. What he needed was encouragement, reassurance, and his question answered in a civil and courteous manner each time.

Do not treat residents as though they were inanimate objects.

Treat people like people, not pieces of furniture. People have feelings, curiosity, preferences, and desires for recognition.

We know when we are being taken for granted, used, or not seen as a real person. Residents know this too. It is diminishing. It shows in how we address them, how we use or don't use their names, and the way we touch or don't touch them. Do we really give personal care?

Call them by their preferred names, appreciate their essence, and touch them with kindness and sincerity.

Do not use sarcasm.

Sometimes we express our feelings of disapproval through exaggeration and hyperbole.

Mr. EE refused to attend any activities. Rather than blurt out an abrupt no he always made excuses. One nursing assistant said to another, "He has so many social engagements." The message and the tone of voice conveyed sarcasm. Mr. EE was crushed.

Sarcasm is a witty release for our frustrations but a devastating put down for the recipient of the verbal thrust.

Do not be too rigid.

Right and wrong, black and white, make for a rigid environment and non-negotiable rules. Granted, fire regulations and other health and safety factors cannot be compromised, but most procedures and policies can take the individual into consideration. Try to remember that most regulations are not written in concrete. People should be more of a priority than rules. If we are willing to negotiate, it lets the residents know that everyone's needs are important. Everyone includes us.

Do not criticize.

This is not to say that residents do not act in ways that are never to be criticized. This is only to say that there are better ways to do it. When we criticize we tell persons that they should not be who they are. We label them. We tend to use words such as always and never, even though we know this absolute cannot be true. Criticizing gives the residents no option on how to change behavior. Conversely, if the behavior is described and we explain how we feel about it we let the residents know that they can choose to behave differently. We refrain from giving them a negative label.

Do not neglect.

Neglect does not necessarily mean that anyone is engaging in any active abuse against the residents. I am not referring to neglect that results in health or safety problems. I am writing about the garden variety neglect in which we give the residents the message that they do not exist, that our time and duties are important and they are not. This is the neglect people feel when we fulfill our needs at the residents' expense. It doesn't make them feel very good about themselves.

Do not over-indulge.

Yes, be supportive. To be sure, we want to give residents special attention and privileges. We do not want to be patronizing and sticky. Over-indulgence makes the residents dependent on us and keeps them dependent. They do not develop as best they can and they do not develop self esteem. This behavior allows us to be needed, but does not address the residents' needs to feel like a separate entity.

Let Them Do What They Can Do

Generally, people know their capabilities. We can't all do everything, but we all can do something. Perhaps that something we can do is contingent upon our receiving help. For example, no astronauts could blast off for the moon without a team to assist, check, and even help dress them. I couldn't drive to work unless someone else knew how to keep the car running. The nursing home residents may be able to wash themselves if someone gets them into the shower. They may be able to pick out their clothes, but not put them on.

Even if physically impaired the nursing home residents can use their minds. They may want to keep track of and discuss their medication. This gives them some control over their environment and a concept of ability. They want to be treated as though they have good sense. They can make choices and offer opinions and observations. If they are treated as though they don't know what they are talking about self esteem will plunge.

Just letting the nursing home residents do what they can do may not be enough. Encouragement is helpful, reinforcing, and can nudge people off center and ahead.

Sometimes nursing home residents will identify a staff job as one that they can do such as filling ice pitchers, calling bingo numbers, orienting new residents, or any number of helpful tasks. Some have to be asked to perform, other will volunteer. They or their contribution should never be expected, tolerated, or patronized. They deserve and should expect thanks and appreciation. They will see their participation as an asset to their living situation. Their self esteem will be increased.

Power

Residents feel better about themselves when they have some power. In our own work and play we get most discomfited when we are bereft of any power to be a participant in what happens to us. We don't like the boss changing the rules and procedures when it involves our job and effects us. We want to be consulted and considered. We need to feel in some control over our lives or all seems to be chaos.

We are all dissimilar and we all exert our power in different ways. We should allow the residents to express their efforts towards power in a constructive way. The stubborn, uncooperative, passive, or aggressive residents are showing their power, but not in a way that is helpful to them or to us.

Ms. FF was a nursing home resident who was respected by others. She respected herself too. She took responsibility for what happened to her in her environment. She took action and used her power when she felt it was necessary. When she saw occurrences that were against rules, regulations, or human dignity, she called the nursing home ombudsman. The committee would always investigate and often changes in procedures were made. Ms. FF rightfully took credit for all improvements. This action did not make Ms. FF the most popular of the nursing home residents, but it earned her esteem.

In one nursing home it was announced that a popular resident meeting and greeting area was going to be turned into a much needed office. The resident group was devastated and attacked the problem with downcast mumbling. A visitor to the home, overhearing their distress, said, "Why don't you picket?" Their attitude changed. They had purpose. They obtained materials from the Activity Department, made signs, and had a sit in. The administrator was so impressed with their intense feelings and assertions that they were allowed to keep their sitting room. They felt power, the satisfaction of a job well done, and increased self esteem.

Ms. GG was elected to represent her wing of the nursing home in the Resident Council. To her this was not a sinecure. She immediately took her duties to heart and supervised care, heard complaints, and reported all infractions. Many staff members felt she was far too enthusiastic about her job and a real pain besides. Nonetheless, Ms. GG persevered and overcame objections. She used her power judiciously and felt great in her elected role.

GENERAL APPROACHES

Support and Encouragement

Giving loving care conveys the message that we care and that the residents needs are important. It is comforting and helpful to the resident. Loving care recognizes the residents as important beings.

Giving support also gives comfort and love. It lets the residents know that we encourage them to think and do for themselves whatever they are able to do. It gives the message that they are capable. It lets the residents know that if they are doing well, someone cares enough to help them do better.

On the other hand, do not be too quick to reassure. Listen first. If we say, "Everything will be fine," or "You'll do all right," before we hear the problem they will know that we do not care enough to really listen. They will also think that they and their problems are unimportant.

Support is significant in helping us be what we can be. So is praise. Praise lights up our lives. Even though overly lavish praise is not effective because it sounds insincere, we do not praise enough. Praise can be given for:

1. Improvement
2. Thoughtfulness
3. Doing the decent thing
4. Appearance
5. Ability
6. Anything at all – anytime at all.

Praise can be given repetitiously, again and again, often, indefinitely, and it always falls on welcoming ears.

Ms. HH was uneasy as she had reported that her roommate had hit another resident. She felt she had made trouble for herself and was torn between looking out for the protection of others and fear of retaliation. Ms. HH was given praise for doing her civic duty while having her confidentiality guarded. Finding that she was seen as behaving in a responsible manner did her self esteem a world of good.

Treat everyone as though they had good self esteem. Persons with self confidence give off an aura that demands respect. Act as though everyone radiates this and give them this regard.

We should be conscious of the nonverbal messages people send out. Some of us want physical closeness and reach out for people. Others want physical distance and appear more standoffish. Some are jokers. Others are serious. Read the signals. Tune in to individual differences and desires. People feel better about themselves when their boundaries are recognized and accepted.

Names

Nicknames can have real meaning. They symbolize the affection family and friends have for the persons by bestowing special names on them. Residents may prefer their nicknames to their given names. The nickname is tied up in their own esteem. They want their nickname used as this is how they think of themselves. Some people have never had a nickname and fancy a more formal approach when addressed. Some have always wanted a nickname and will respond positively to an affectionate and respectful one awarded them by their caregivers. A nickname that says something positive can be used. Demeaning nicknames should be avoided. Do not even think in terms of crybaby, whiner, pincher, sourpuss, or other degrading designations. The nickname gets in the mind and suggests how the individuals should be treated. One nursing home employee called a resident Snuggles and gave her a hug whenever she saw her. The resident responded and began to expect this pleasant interaction. Her facial expression became happier and happier. This was a positive nickname for the resident. It may have been a belittling one for another. The nickname must fit people's concept of themselves. To go against this is to go against self esteem. Some nicknames confer praise and recognition when they tie in a fact about the resident with an affectionate title such as calling the woman from Georgia a Georgia Peach, or the retired New York policeman, New York's Finest.

Use whatever name the residents' prefer. The emphasis is on the name. They do not want to be called he/she, lady, or you. We have names so we can be differentiated from others. Our name is part of our status and self esteem. We like to hear it and have others remember it. The sound of our name spoken with affection or recognition always brings us pleasure.

Special Attention

To have good self esteem residents should have the freedom to do whatever they want to do as long as it doesn't hurt anyone. This is a basic philosophy that should permeate a nursing home.

Families should be encouraged to take their loved ones out to lunch, to their home, or to special events as long as the residents' health is taken into consideration. There is an element of pride that comes from having someplace to go and to be able to return and tell our friends about it. Part of the pleasure of an experience is being able to share it. We should listen to the residents describe the events, show interest, and let them know they are special to have been a participant. Another part of an outing is the self esteem accrued from having been invited and of knowing that there are people who desire their company.

If the residents can't go home goodies from home mean a lot. Again this reflects on esteem. If we get more from others we interpret it to mean that we are worth more. Food is nice, but pictures, handcrafted items, any article that helps with show and tell are effective. Videos of family occasions, with a narration that includes how much the resident was missed, can be excellent for the spirits.

Ms. II developed a good relationship with the nurse on the day shift. They could talk. They listened to each other. Occasionally the nurse would bring Ms. II food she cooked that she thought would be enjoyable. Ms. II was thrilled and rewarded the nurse with sparkling appreciation. The nurse's self esteem soared. Ms. II's self esteem was also raised because she was singled out for special attention.

During the course of everyday events humorous incidents come up. At work and with our families in-jokes develop. These in-jokes contribute to a sense of belonging and inclusion.

Nursing homes are rich with material for in-jokes. Every resident knows of one staff member who has had an embarrassing moment that turned out to be funny. The time the exercise leader pointed to her shoulders and meant her feet has been an ongoing in-joke for the exercise class. When the new nursing assistant, who didn't know the residents, tried to help militantly independent Mr. JJ take a bath an ongoing chuckle was born. Mr. JJ laughs whenever anyone kids him about being ready to help him with his ablutions.

Staff members should be able and willing to laugh at themselves. It is good for morale and being part of a humorous incident is good for individual self esteem.

Mr. KK and the nursing home administrator had their own in-joke. They both recall the time she decided to deliver a bouquet to his room and ended up dropping it at his bedside. After a moment of horror and quick picking up and rearranging they could both release the tension in hilarity. Her grace in being the butt of a joke and his in seeing the humor in a potential disaster gave them a relationship that bound them together in an easy comraderie. Mr. KK felt pretty good about himself too since he had this special tie to the administrator.

Included in laughing at ourselves is admitting mistakes. The nursing home residents know that they make plenty of them. It helps their self esteem to know that other people make mistakes too. When they can make light of them it helps them to dismiss their own blunders and still feel good about themselves.

Of course, we cannot laugh at every mishap. But we can own up to errors, apologize for them, and try to make amends. This all adds to the residents' acceptance of self. They feel as though they are being treated as worthwhile people when they are shown these honest courtesies.

Friendships

When many people live in close proximity we worry about cliques, not because it is not good for those who join them, but because it can look like favoritism and the shutting out of others.

Let's try to look at this phenomenon from a more positive viewpoint. Choosing our own friends is a decided right in our lives. Even as children we didn't like our parents to tell us with whom we should play. As adults we would not want to be put back into that position. We encourage friendships among nursing home residents. It enlarges and enhances the quality of their life. Having good social relationships elevates health and happiness.

Friendship needs nearness and time to develop. People have to be able to see each other regularly over a period of time to have a relationship go beyond social niceties to an emotional closeness. This means that residents who have friendships should have rooms in the same hallway and be allowed to eat together. The frail elderly cannot pursue an association with someone if it takes too much energy for them to travel to be near the person.

When the atmosphere in a nursing home is such that it encourages close relationships and the environment makes it possible, groups of residents will develop a close community from which they will draw status and satisfaction.

Ms. LL was never thrilled with nursing home living. Her entire life had been made up of coffee parties, luncheons, and social interchanges with a group of long time friends. They loved to talk about their children, their husbands, and their day to day lives. That all changed with the nursing home admission. The only joy in her living arrangements seemed to be when one of her former associates took her out for coffee. She lived from one such occasion to the next. They did not occur often as her friends were elderly too. This all changed when they became nursing home residents. She could feel good about herself again because she and her friends met regularly to talk and snack together. All went well. They were happy and animated until the nursing home staff said they could no longer group together for coffee and cookies as it looked as though they were getting special treatment. Ms. LL wilted. She grumbled. She took to meeting her friends secretly. It was never the same. Her pleasure in her life and in herself did not regain its former level.

The Little Things

All of us have tendencies to gravitate to certain people. Just as we are different in our choice of friends, so do we have our own idiosyncracies. We can maintain our eccentricities because we live in our own households and have the independence to do so. We wouldn't want to give them up (or even be able to) just because we had to change our life style from separate to communal living. Think about this when a resident insists that her clock stays set on standard time, refusing to switch to daylight savings. Have consideration for the resident who is obdurate that her television stay on channel five. Help Ms. MM into her corset. Let Ms. NN wear her once fashionable suit. Be sure Mr. OO never has one thing on his bedside stand rearranged. Straighten Mr. PP's pictures. Don't insist that it doesn't make any difference if Ms. QQ has a blue or a red lap robe. It does to her. These are not trivial matters. They have important psychological consequences. There is no point in causing unnecessary distress. Doing so worsens the residents' condition and self esteem.

Helping the Residents Be Helpful

A measure of our self esteem is tied up in our contribution to others. We become nonpersons when we have nothing to give. Even if we can only give a smile or respond with a look of comfort we are giving back to those who give to us. It is what we get back from what we are doing (over and above the pay check) that keeps us doing it. The nursing home residents need to be in a position to give. They need to have appreciation and the feeling of a job well done. Some residents manage to achieve this on their own. Ms. RR crochets and hands out pot holders. Ms. SS tells jokes. Mr. TT always has candy on hand to share. Other residents are so overwhelmed in a new environment that they need help to find a place where they can contribute. We can let them know when they say or do something that makes our day. We can point out what their smile or comfort means to us. It is in our power to let them hear how much we appreciate their comments, their feedback.

Giving Suggestions

Help the residents give verbally. Ask for and encourage their opinions. We need not pressure them to state their case, but we don't need to give up too easily either. When they learn that we are really interested and will accept their point of view, even if it differs from ours, they will become more willing to enrich our lives with their ideas and observations. Knowing their opinion counts is tremendous for their self esteem.

Go from soliciting opinions to asking for suggestions. If it is totally unwarranted explain why it can't be used. If suggestions are ignored, they will stop coming. Listen and learn. What may seem far fetched may have an element of merit.

Ms. UU did not like being out of sight of her room because she would get disoriented and feel insecure about finding her way back. Nevertheless, she wanted to attend weekly church services. They were held in a dining room on another hall. She suggested that they be held alternate weeks in her regular dining area. This was dismissed as too confusing and jokingly shared with the minister. The pastor liked the idea, but modified it to having two shorter services, one in each wing of the nursing home. This increased church attendance as it made it feasible for more residents to attend. The minister gave Ms. UU a written commendation for her suggestion. She glowed with pride.

Giving Assistance

Some people have formed a life time habit of being useful to others. They want to continue this. Give them the opportunity and encouragement to do so. Others need a little push to see the benefit of being of use to others. Program them in that direction by identifying what they can do to help others and praising them when they do. A few of the things residents can do for others are:

1. Call for assistance.
2. Give directions.
3. Give information.
4. Invite to activities or events.
5. Share treats.
6. Get water or ice.
7. Help locate belongings.
8. Make introductions.
9. Welcome to the facility, area, room.
10. Explain procedures.
11. Write cards or letters.
12. Read mail or papers.
13. Assist in games.
14. Visit the sick or bed bound.
15. Report problems.

Being useful gives the residents a niche in the scheme of things and adds to their esteem.

Our attitude can maximize the residents' abilities, contributions, and self esteem.

Ms. VV was a retired social worker suffering from painful and disabling arthritis. She was cantankerous and unreasonable most of the time. No one knew how to handle her, or wanted to. She was impossible to please. The nursing home social worker continued unswerving support. She helped her with her social security problems. She negotiated family visits. She managed to entice her on some facility outings. Her disposition didn't change, but a relationship developed between Ms. VV and the social worker. Ms. VV became conscious of the social worker's needs and noted one day that she seemed depressed. By way of explanation the social worker mentioned that she was having trouble with her daughter. What happened from there on seemed a miracle. Ms. VV's experience, training, and honest desire to assist her own helper surged forth. She gave of herself and her knowledge and was of inestimable value to the nursing home social worker. She gave support and insight. She was there when needed and knew she was valued and appreciated. She felt useful! Her attitude towards herself changed and her behavior towards others moderated. She liked herself again. This showed in what appeared as a total personality change. She was less suspicious, less querulous, and more open and giving. She became popular!

This example is not to encourage staff to take their problems to the residents for help. It is given to show that using one's abilities and being needed can make one feel great. If the social worker had not had a long standing relationship with the resident she would not have burdened her with her personal problems. She did so only because they had already been through so much together and had developed a personal as well as a professional relationship.

We also see from this example that a job that fits one's skills is enhancing to self esteem. With this in mind it is ever so wonderful to find tasks for residents that relate to their self concepts, their interests, their past work experiences, and their physical abilities. This is a tall order, but it does not have to be career oriented or full time. Sometimes it will give the residents enough satisfaction to just make their own beds. Some residents find reward in raising the flag, others in distributing the mail. Ms. WW attached herself to the Activity Department and made it her job to take attendance at every event. This was a valuable contribution, for which she was frequently thanked and praised.

Doing a worthwhile job does give us self satisfaction, but to really feel good about ourselves we need to know that others see our contribution as significant too. We want to hear it. Over time we need reinforcement that we are still appreciated and important.

Never allow anyone to take on an overwhelming, overly ambitious piece of work. Nor should too much be assigned or requested. If the residents see the task as too much for them they are defeated before they begin. It feels hopeless to start. Break any task into small parts so it can be accomplished a step at a time, or several can work on it at once or in phases. When there are manageable steps the goals appear possible. Achievement is balm to the ego.

Residents working together or with staff provide another esteem enhancing opportunity. This sets up the occasion for sharing. There is a chance to share work, thoughts, feelings, histories, experiences, and day to day happenings that build trust, caring, and regard for self and others.

Ms. XX was friendly and helpful. However, she was secretive and did not share her personal life with anyone. She avoided all activities that had to do with reminiscing, autobiography, or any self revelation. She was an active participant in ceramics. It was during this regularly scheduled event that she was able to talk more easily about herself. The ceramics teacher did not probe. She was always accepting and shared both facts and feelings. It was through this experience that Ms. XX learned self acceptance, became less guarded, and was able to be more free around others. She came to the point where all of her could be esteemed, rather than just the parts of her she had chosen to let others see.

Being Attractive

Personal appearance is a small segment of any person. Even so, we spend a lot of time on how we look. Fortunes are made on products that can improve our physical attractiveness. Obviously we pay attention to the features viewed by the public.

Clothes, hair styles, makeup, good grooming and compliments are crucial. Ordinary care and attention should manage the above. We need to go a step beyond and protect the residents with physical problems from personal embarrassment. This does not mean that we keep them from the public eye. This means that we help them be acceptable and admirable while with others.

A common problem in nursing homes is incontinence. Residents can be mortified by these uncontrollable incidents. Subtly, quietly, and with every effort to help the residents keep their self respect, their needs should be handled. Heroic steps must be taken to keep people dry, looking and smelling good, and thus, feeling good.

Other physical difficulties that result in drooling and spilling food should be monitored with vigilance so that physical attractiveness is marred as little as possible. Always keep in mind how much our society values neatness and cleanliness and how these values are wrapped up in our self esteem. The residents depend on us to keep these values intact for them.

One sure way we know we are attractive is if someone of the opposite sex is enamored with us. Even if not interested in romance, attention from an admirer is fun and does wonders for our self esteem. Make it possible for interaction among men and women so that they can exhibit gallantry and find pleasure in each other.

Chapter III

SELF ESTEEM ENHANCEMENT PROGRAMS

So far we have discussed approaches, attitudes, and atmosphere within the nursing home that may enhance the residents' self esteem. In this section we will deal with actual ongoing programs and activities that contribute to enriched self esteem.

BACKGROUND STATEMENT

Most of everything written in this book, before and what follows, is known and is being done. The message is clear, keep it up! The other emphasis is for us to know why what we are doing is good for self esteem. When we realize the portent of our contributions it may help our own self esteem! We have noticed that activities make people behave with more animation and zest. The reason is not only that the residents have taken an interest in life, but more importantly, have taken an interest in themselves. We are the ones that have made that possible. We have provided the vehicle that gets them back on the path to a happy, fulfilling life.

Many of the programs are simple. They are so simple as to seem simplistic. Such is not the case. They have shown results. Not everyone responds to everything. Everybody gives a response to something. Some work immediately for some people. Some people need constant and continual reinforcement. Some respond only after a long period of time in an ongoing program. Although the approach is one minded, enhancing self esteem, the results differ as do the people, depending on the various personality components, their experiences, and their own personal characteristics. Since none of the suggested activities will harm anyone they can all be tried. If they don't help the residents' self esteem they may help them pass the time, have some fun, and interact with others. We have nothing to lose, as we will be doing our jobs while we are enriching individual lives. We will be the catalyst for rewarding experiences.

Some of the projects described will be suited for confused residents, others for the more alert and oriented. Almost all can be adapted for use with both.

Whenever applicable the endeavor should be ongoing so that the residents have a goal to work towards. This gives life purpose. It becomes achievement oriented. It makes all things more possible.

PROGRAMS FOR INDIVIDUALS

Self esteem should not be for designated times and places. Working on behalf of the residents' self esteem is always and forever. Nor should certain staff members be assigned self esteem duties. This is a job for everyone working in concert.

Feeling Good Programs

Identifying Good Times

Help the residents identify feel good times. If they can't tell us of incidents of contentment, notice when they seem the happiest. Some residents find their best time is the morning. Others get their greatest pleasure in meals. There are residents who are only content when they are occupied or entertained. Emphasize these times with them. Let them know what they do that brings satisfaction. This will bring them more enjoyment. They will concentrate more on the positive aspects of their day. They will feel as though life is worth living and the time they put into it is of value.

Letting Go

When residents are cranky it is often due to something unpleasant that occurred earlier in the day. They have kept the thought and/or feeling and let it gnaw away in their minds. They can also feel happy for no apparent reason. I'm sure we agree that it is much better to have the happy than the dismal. Take time to help them identify the origin of these feelings. Once we have taught them how, they can do it for themselves. They will be able to recapture and dwell on the good feelings and deal with and dismiss the wretched ones. Use the following technique.

Have the residents close their eyes and think back through their day. Start them with the morning hours. Say:

"It is 6:00 A.M. Think about the people around you. Think how they acted. What did they say? What were their expressions? How did you act? How did you feel? Remember all that happened. Hold on to the good things, the things you liked, those that made you happy. Let go of any unpleasant feeling or trans- action. It is past. You cannot change it now."

"It is now 9:00 A.M. to noon. Who were you with? What did you do? How did you feel? Keep everything pleasant and let the offensive go. It is past. You cannot change it now."

"It is noon to 2:00 P.M. How are you feeling? How do you look? How do you act? What are people around you doing? What are the sights? The sounds? The smells? Remember what's fun. Get rid of the displeasing. Let it go. It is past. You cannot change it now."

Continue to take them through their day until they determine their point of dissatisfaction or find the delightful portions that they want to cherish. We can start at any part of the day and go by minutes, hours, or sections. The point is to remember, to let go, and to move on. This is a particularly good exercise at night as it contributes to relaxed, untroubled sleep and a complacent feeling in the morning.

It is effective to do the exercise along with the residents, speaking in the first person. We find it ameliorative for staff and residents alike. As we rethink our day, we can rearrange our thoughts, feelings, and reactions and convey the positive result to the residents. When they see how the process helps us they will feel more inspired to use it for their own purposes.

This exercise lets us know how much control we really have over what happens to us. We can create our own day by how we react to people and events.

Catch Them Doing Good

Take the opportunity to help residents feel good about themselves, identify the best times in their day, and at the same time mold appropriate behavior. Catch them doing right. We don't want to praise people for doing what is considered unpraiseworthy or to give them false compliments just to help their self esteem. Nor do we want to encourage residents to feel good about behavior that is dangerous to themselves or others. We want to help them know when they are handling themselves in a way that can make them proud and is also admired by others. When they do this, even if they don't see it as the high spot of their day, point it out to them. Don't stop there. Praise them. Tell others about the great deed they did. Refer back to it throughout the day or week. We caught them doing something that should give them self respect and was helpful. It was something they could feel good about. Let them know the many positive rewards that accrue to that kind of behavior.

Self Affirmations

When we were growing up we didn't always get unqualified approval. Church, school, relatives, and neighbors all seemed to conspire to teach us to do right by giving us negatives. We were told what not to do, and told that often. It certainly was pointed out to us what we did that was wrong. Throughout life we have carried these do nots with us and had them reinforced in employment situations when our bosses only gave us attention when we didn't do quite right.

Nursing home residents are no different from the rest of us. We all have our minds cluttered with negative messages that start with the phrases:

I can't.

I shouldn't.

I'm not.

In essence we are telling ourselves that we are unable, unlikable, and unworthy. We have the opportunity to turn these messages around with self affirmations. We can give the residents self affirmations. They can learn to do this for themselves, erasing the negative tapes they carry in their brains, and replacing them with:

I can.

I will.

I am.

The method is effective, but deceptively simple. All residents will need follow up on their progress as they will consider it foolish, embarrassing, and ineffective. It is so easy to do, yet so difficult, because it is hard to praise ourselves, even to ourselves.

This magical method involves writing down and memorizing five or six phrases geared towards enhancing our self esteem. We say these to ourselves each morning and every evening. That is all there is to it. What is there to lose? We should be able to convince residents to try something that takes so little effort, even if they are skeptical about the results. They should begin to feel the effects of their own positive statements in about two weeks. Even though they will feel better about themselves this soon, they should be told to continue their self affirmations on a daily basis. Some suggested self affirmations for self esteem are:

I am likeable.

I am capable.

I am attractive.

I am worthy.

Every day in every way I am getting better and better.

These general positive statements apply to anyone. We might help the residents add one or two that apply specifically to them, such as statements that recognize positive qualities they already possess. They might be:

I am a good friend.

I have a great smile.

I am giving.

I am caring.

People admire me.

Always check the residents' affirmative statements before they start using them to make sure no negative element slips in. In our culture we are not accustomed to self aggrandizement. It is easy to qualify the positives by saying:

Most people like me.

I often do right.

I am good at some things.

Do not allow this. As much as we admire modesty, this is not the time or the place for it. All self affirmations must be absolutely, completely, and unqualifiably positive.

Ms. YY, a lovely lady in her eighties, was always putting herself down. She said she was old, in the way, made mistakes, did the wrong things, and was quick to respond with an "I can't," whenever asked to do anything. When her abilities were pointed out to her she would shrug them off, even though it was apparent she liked the reassurance. It was suspected that she was so verbal about her failings just so she could hear someone else tell her that it wasn't really true. The nursing assistant suggested that Ms. YY try self affirmations so that she could discover her own fine qualities. She found it impossible to think of anything good about herself. The nursing assistant, undeterred, made a list that included:

I am pretty.

I am worthwhile.

I can do anything.

People like me.

She gave Ms. YY the list and kept one herself. Each morning she asked the resident if she had said her self affirmations. Ms. YY would regularly reply, "No, I can't do that." The nursing assistant would then say them to her and encourage her to try. After two weeks Ms. YY stopped protesting. It took another two weeks for her to start on her own. In a month and a half Ms. YY was invited to join the facility newspaper staff. She replied, "I can do that. I used to write in high school." The staff was thrilled and praised both Ms. YY and her nursing assistant. She was encouraged to continue her self affirmations. Now and then the nursing assistant would say them with her. She no longer appeared disconcerted by them.

Appreciation Day

There is something we can appreciate in even the most odious of people. Make it a habit to tell them. Set the stage so residents may do the same. In fact, a formalized appreciation day isn't a bad idea. During this day everyone tells everyone else one thing they appreciate about that person. It may be a small thing, such as the resident eats well, doesn't cry out at night, or gets up willingly. We can mention their looks or grooming. It can even be a compliment about their friends or relatives. Or it can be more personal and relate to the way they treat others. Appreciation day gets icky if done too often as too much sweetness can make us uncomfortable. It should be scheduled often enough to reinforce the necessity of giving praise to give self esteem, but not so often that we groan and say, "Not again!" A quarterly appreciation day is probably about right.

Responding for Positive Feedback

Be a teacher. Teach residents to give responses or make comments that brings them positive feedback. This is easier for some than others. Using appreciation day to show that they get thanks and smiling attention for saying nice things is a good beginning. Giving the resident time or something they may want such as a treat or some special assistance also lets them know that there are rewards in saying kind words.

Mr. ZZ was a grouch and only spoke when he wanted something, unless he got on the topic of the Bible. His knowledge was impressive, but his interpretation was so individual as to seem bizarre. Whenever Mr. ZZ would ask for something in a pleasant way or would talk about any topic other than the Bible his nursing assistant would allow him time, give him attention, and listen to him talk a few minutes on his biblical beliefs. He soon learned that when he was agreeable, he got better feedback from other people. His behavior slowly changed from barely sufferable to tolerable. (Hey, don't expect miracles.)

Written Messages of Good Will

Verbal appreciation is terrific. Sometimes more is needed. An effective tool to enhance self esteem is to write down the residents' good traits or abilities. When residents are feeling low give them a note saying that they are good at crocheting, singing, telling jokes, smiling, winking, or anything you can think of that is true. In some instances a list of their superior qualities can be made and posted for them to see. This is not like a self affirmation when they are trying to change their attitude about themselves. These are written confirmations of what is good and right and recognized by others.

See the Happiness

No matter how bad things seem, help the residents learn to count their blessings each morning. There is a danger in this approach. There may be a tendency to discount the residents concerns, complaints, and very real distress. These need to be acknowledged. The next step is to help the residents see that all is not bleak. The sun is up. They have someone to care for them. Their relatives visit. They can talk, read, write, play cards, watch television, or whatever they can do and enjoy. Always emphasize that there is still something for which they can be thankful. When things look the darkest we need someone to remind us of the light. This doesn't dispel what is troubling us, but does get us away from tunnel vision. It also helps us feel a little better about our lives.

Strength Mottos

Post a motto in the residents' rooms. Give them a selection or have them come up with their own that gives inspiration and accentuates self esteem. Some suggestions are:

You are a star!

You can do anything!

You're a winner!

You're No. 1!

You are my favorite person!

This is a passive way to work on self esteem. The message is always there.

Can You Top This?

Get the residents to give fantastic and superlative answers when they are asked how they are. Most often the how are you question is purely social and no one really wants to know the details of people's physical and emotional health. When someone needs to know they can answer specifically and factually. Otherwise they can say fine. However, this is hardly colorful enough. They can learn from us to say they are terrific, invincible, or on top of the world! If we are OK, they can be super! If they are the best ever, we can be sensational! Get out the dictionary and try to top each other with fabulous and stupendous adjectives. It makes a person feel better just to use such extravagant words.

Comments to Visitors

It helps the residents' self esteem to hear us praise them to visiting friends and relatives. My aunt, who has never had a self esteem problem, but like all of us needs little boosts now and then, was pleased to report that the activity assistant had told visiting friends, in her presence, that she made an important contribution to the program as she always had something interesting to add. At age ninety four it is fulfilling to continue to be a valued participant. Try to keep some complimentary tidbits in mind that can be reported to kith or kin when the residents can hear what is being said. It does not have to be a momentous earth shaking gem, but it must be sincere.

Comparisons

Comparisons are usually not to our liking unless they are flattering. We enjoy complimentary comparisons. It is fun to hear that we remind someone of their best friend, favorite teacher, or a loved member of their own family. We are not averse to hearing that we look like a famous and attractive celebrity or that we share some characteristics of a notable person. We don't mind hearing that we are as smart as some brilliant personality or have a sense of humor as good as a great comedian's. It is the unfavorable comparison or the comparison that is used to try to make us change our behavior that is loathsome. It is easy to get a smile and a thank you from any of us when we are told that we conjure up a memory of someone we like and revere. Comparisons to our own relatives, if we have high regard for them, also makes us feel better about ourselves.

Individual Attention

Special Events

When we do or attend something special we feel pretty special ourselves. Just getting outside the facility to go to church can be a red letter event for residents who have no other opportunities to leave the nursing home. One resident was able to eat out at a fast food restaurant and put a bumper sticker on her wheelchair that advertised the chain. Another, who was invited to a nursing assistant's home for dinner still talked about the occasion a year later, describing the family and their reactions to her.

There is status in doing something that everyone else doesn't get to do. The group that went to the zoo raved about the animals. The picnickers thought the modest fare they had to eat was the best meal they had tasted in ages. The few residents who got to be in the local parade felt as though they had been elected president, monarch, and prime minister all at one time. Since they were able to do special things they felt as though they were special people. Pictures of the event helped them recapture the excitement and enabled them to show others.

Family Events

Ms. AB had her nephew from Germany visit her everyday for a week. This gave her status and attention as everybody was interested in him and then in her life in Germany before she came to this country. A part of her life that was long gone now became an element in her self esteem.

Mr. BC's granddaughter married in another state. Her parents sent a video of the event. He invited friends to view the wedding with him. It became a special occasion he could share.

Residents love to tell about visits to the family home and focus on what interests them. Some describe the food. Others talk about their grandchildren. The financial or career accomplishments are the emphasis of a few. Material possessions may also be highlighted. Being with their families is a symbol of being wanted and does a lot for the residents' self esteem. When we express interest and listen to a review of the event we are enhancing their self esteem.

Encourage families to make the nursing home resident as much a part of their lives as is feasible. If the trip is too far, too long, or too tiring try to have them include the resident with pictures, videos, or mementos. If the resident can't leave the nursing home perhaps the family can make a point of bringing the family affair to the resident.

Ms. CD did not remember well, but she always recalled her last birthday. On that date, at her daughter's home, her grandson pinned a badge on her that said, "World's Best Grandmother." She wore this everywhere and always received smiles, congratulations, and inquiries regarding it. She was always reminded of the esteem of her family.

Remembered Events

Our memories are a vital and important part of our being. It is an emotional experience to review the circumstances of our lives that made us what we are today. Residents find that discussing their past in relationship to something that is going on currently gives them self esteem. This is because they can be seen as multidimensional persons. Nursing home residents sometimes are seen as old, dependent, without past or future, and needing the care the staff can give them. Instead they have intriguing observations on the passing scene based on incidents in their own lives.

Residents remember awards, honors, and significant events and feel pride in sharing them. Their self esteem is rekindled as they talk about promotions, graduations, honorable discharges, retirements, school attainments, or anything that has brought them special recognition. These are common occurrences in people's lives and can be a part of daily conversations. They hope to gain our esteem by telling of their successes. They will advance their own esteem by doing so.

Talking with someone who accepts us, no matter what, also helps us accept ourselves. Each of us has elements in our makeup that make us less than proud and lowers our self esteem. The goal in self esteem is to accept all of ourselves. We may not like everything we do, feel, or have done, but it is all part of us. When the residents talk about the matters that may have embarrassed or disappointed them, and have them accepted and understood by someone they trust, it is possible for them to see themselves in a better light. Remembering helps them get out the secrets, become a whole person, and feel totally acceptable.

Memories can be triggered by possessions. An article of clothing or a picture may remind the residents of special events in their lives, either fondly recalled or tinged with remorse or sorrow. Ms. DE spent time alone and also with ds and family going through her jewelry box. As she ched the ornaments she told about the time, the place, and e people each item brought to mind. In this way she was able to put her life in perspective.

These memories are not the common reminiscences many of us have of the times in which we were raised such as the economics, fashion, and equipment of the era. The remembered events referred to here are specific to the individuals and are affirmations of their lives.

Imaginary Trips

We can escape anytime we want. We can make mental trips. This is a special sort of remembering in which people can go anywhere they want at any time.

Residents can pick special people or places for their imaginary trips. They can even go somewhere they've never been before. They can be a part of reconstructed or totally imagined events. It is their chance to have everything just as they had hoped it was or could be. It is like a daydream with them as the major actors. They can be the heros, the stars, the people in charge. To relive an actual event is fun. To imagine the self being in the central role is good for self esteem.

Volunteer Work

Volunteer work takes the residents out of themselves and their environment and lets them know that they are valued by others in their community. Besides getting positive feedback from the people they work with, they will receive awards, plaques, and written commendations. Sometimes there are writeups in the newspaper or blurbs on radio and television. It all helps self esteem.

There is no end to volunteer work in the community. Even in very small towns there are usually schools and churches. Children need tutoring. Churches need paper work such as folding, stuffing, and mailing. The Council on Aging not only has work suited to the individual, but regularly scheduled meetings to attend to give the resident a sense of belonging. There are residents who like to work for and attend meetings related to their own disease, such as arthritis or stroke clubs.

Volunteering can take place within the facility. Depending on the residents' interests and abilities they can work in various departments, with individuals, or with groups. There is always clerical work in administration. Dietary must need someone to do a survey now and then. Housekeeping can use the services of a puddle patrol. Activities and Social Services can put individuals into one to one contact with bedridden residents. There may be individuals who can lead groups. The Nursing Department can use supervised assistance for routine work.

Recognition for all volunteer work is crucial. Busy work is OK if it satisfies a need. It is not OK if the person gets no appreciation or satisfaction.

If residents are unable to volunteer physically, they may be able to volunteer information or possessions. Ms. EF, a retired newspaper reporter, subscribed to four newspapers. She was proud to have her papers borrowed and selected stories read during residents' news time. She started to specify items of particular general interest and reveled in the contribution she made.

Special Privileges

The regimen and the schedules are what bugs many nursing home residents. If only they could have coffee at 8:00 P.M., go to bed at midnight, and sleep until 10:00 A.M. they would feel like real people. Nursing home staff cannot cater to all idiosyncratic needs, but when allowances can be made, the residents feel like special people, indeed. Ms. FG was honored to be allowed to smoke in the bookkeeper's office

(She smoked too.). Mr. GH enjoyed the privilege of helping himself to coffee from the nursing staff's pot. Ms. HI liked having tea with her nursing assistant.

Special Possessions

Ms. HI had some religious tapes. They were very special to her. She selected people to hear them. It made her feel important that she could furnish this opportunity to her friends and certain staff members. Everyone learned that her ego was tied up in the tapes and their use.

Ms. IJ had a lap size keyboard. The chance to go to the Activity room daily and practice this musical instrument gave her the status she needed. In the meantime her keyboard was much admired and her progress noted. There is no question but that this made her day!

Mr. JK had a mylar balloon tied to his wheelchair. As it deflated his relatives provided him with a new one. The cheerful balloon brought smiles and comments. It became an extension of his personality. He loved it and depended on it to bring him recognition and attention.

Humor

Everybody has a sense of humor. Sometimes it is hard to dredge up. Sometimes it seems impossible to get even a wisp of a smile from a person. But, somewhere in everyone is a funny bone. Use it to help the individual's self esteem. Humor makes people feel good about themselves. It also alleviates stress. It is good for physical and emotional health.

The reason humor has to be individualized is because people find different things funny. I do not particularly enjoy the physical kinds of humor that involve pratfalls, bangs on the head, and pies in the face. Neither do I like ethnic or off color jokes. Some of the residents delight in any or all of the above. Mr. KL did. He was uproarious when I rolled his wheelchair over my foot. That was his kind of good fun. I could laugh with him because I enjoyed the fact that he was having fun. Some residents love puns. Many residents will get a good laugh out of stories that involve the cute sayings of children. Some humor is funny because it is so true to life. Other jokes are laughable because they are so far fetched. Find out what makes the residents laugh. Use their kind of jokes and have a good chuckle together.

Team Work

Working together gives a sense of comraderie, a feeling of sharing, and a sociable perception of congeniality. Not only does it feel good, it makes people feel needed and a critical part of the group. It facilitates the accomplishment of what could otherwise not be completed.

Ms. LM could sew if Ms. MN threaded the needle for her. Mr. NO could do the ceramic glazing, but not the detail work. Ms. OP did that. Mr. PQ gathered news for the facility newspaper and reported it to Mr. QR who wrote it up. Mr. RS typed it in final form. Each belonged to a specific group dedicated to accomplishing an end product. They all contributed. They all were important. They all had enhanced self esteem.

Special Responsibilities

Ms. ST always emptied the ash trays in the dining room. Ms. TU fed the fish. Mr. UV trained the parrot to talk. Mr. VW distributed the newspapers. Mr. WX invited all new residents to activities. Mr. XY gave the weather forecast over the intercom every morning. Mr. YZ made sure each calendar had the right date. The residents knew that they were needed for those particular duties as their jobs were necessary ones. It would be noticed if it were not done. They got attention and esteem.

Awards and Announcements

All the people mentioned in the previous paragraph could appropriately receive awards for services and have an announcement made over the intercom regarding their contribution to the running of the facility. Since they each have a regular job they could be mentioned routinely in the monthly nursing home newsletter.

Stretch your imagination so that recognition can be given to those who might not otherwise receive it. Give an appreciation or achievement sticker to the person with the loudest laugh, the one with the most visitors, or the resident with the brownest eyes. These are meaningful awards. They recognize the special attributes of the individual.

Announcements can concern family members and may be related to milestones such as births, marriages, graduations, and job changes. They can be acknowledged individually with the resident and/or placed in a special section of the facility newsletter. It will induce widespread interest in the publication. It will also enhance the self image of the residents. They will appear as multi-faceted people because of the happenings in the lives of their loved ones.

Awards can be made by the residents too. Let them crown their Valentine King and Queen. Give them the responsibility for presenting the volunteers with their plaques. Help them go out into the community to tender honors on supportive businesses and organizations. It feels important to be the one to endow prestige on another.

Independence

Any program that promotes independence promotes healthy self esteem. Train the residents to do as much for themselves as they can. Make self help tools available to them. Encourage relatives to provide clothing and equipment they can handle themselves.

Dedications

As much as we'd like to be immortal, we can't go on forever. One way to achieve the pretense of perpetuity is to have our names immortalized. We can do this by dedicating something to the individual. People name buildings and businesses after themselves because it makes them feel so good to do so. It gives them pride in themselves and their achievements. We can do the same for the residents, even if it is in a more limited way. Why can't the lobby be named after the resident who always shares flowers and plants by placing them out there for everyone to see? Why can't tables in the dining rooms be named for the residents who occupy them? If residents work extra hard on some project or in some group perhaps the project or the group could be given their name. If something is done in a certain way because a resident wants it that way it can be called the (resident's name) procedure. Bestow the dedications with thoughtfulness — and improvisation.

PROGRAMS FOR GROUPS

Theme Songs and Other Rituals

Groups will be better attended and enjoyed more if the residents see them as a treat, a gathering of friends, or a special event. Not every organized activity can be a stellar happening. Most are on going, regularly scheduled programs. It is these routine affairs that have to have an extra zip to them to help the residents feel good about them and about themselves. One way to do this is to have a theme song or some other ritual suited for each activity. Theme songs give the feeling of belonging, of being one of the "in" people. They need not be original. We might sing any song that is emblazoned on most memories, such as, "For He's a Jolly Good Fellow," "Hail, Hail, the Gang's All Here," or "You Are My Sunshine." One of the residents can be the song leader.

Other rituals for other activities can be discussing the weather, telling a joke, shaking hands, drinking coffee, or eating a cookie. When we become a part of a tradition, we identify with that particular group, and some of our self esteem comes from that identification.

Individual Preferences

Acknowledging individual preferences in the group is marvelous for self esteem. Remember that Ms. ZY likes to sit near the door. Put Mr. YX near the speaker because of his hearing problem. Ms. XW can be seated so that there is no sunlight or glare on her weak eyes. Ms. WV needs a chair with arms because of a balance problem. Mr. VU prefers to sit close to the bathroom. Ms. UT likes her coffee black. We let the residents know that we are aware of their preferences and want to cater to them because they deserve special consideration. This does wonders for their self esteem.

T Shirts and Badges of Belonging

Sports shirts emblazoned with the members' team name were popular long before the present wave of T shirts that advertise our beliefs, make a statement, or express humor. Use this craze for the benefit of the residents' morale and esteem. Issue T shirts for members of the bowling and volley ball teams. T shirts advertising the nursing home serve several purposes. They publicize the facility, give the resident a feeling of being a part of something, and are easy to wear and wash.

If T shirts seem too ambitious a project, or are not suitable for many residents, consider pins, badges, or some kind of personal embellishment (not a tattoo), which indicates membership. This gives the residents another outlet for their self esteem needs.

Resident of the Week

Merit may not be the only reason for selecting a resident of the week. Everyone needs to be somebody. Fame can be awarded by chance. It does not demean the importance of the acknowledgment. One such way is to select the resident of the week through a public drawing. Double honor can be achieved by having one resident draw for the name. After the person has been picked, that name goes into a dormant box until everyone has had their week in the spotlight. New residents' names can be added to the active box. In this way each resident gets to be the special person at least once. Even if the residents are not aware of their distinctive honor the family, friends, staff, and other residents will be. If the facility is particularly large we may want to structure our lottery so that we have a resident of the week from each area of the nursing home.

Just having the drawing and making a public announcement is not enough. More acclaim goes with this event if self esteem is to be maximized. There should be a picture and written profile posted in a well traveled area so that everyone can see the snap and read about the resident. Not only public notice, but obvious favor should be a part of the week long time of glory. The designated resident could be served first in the dining room. The honoree can be asked if she/he has any words of advice for the rest of the residents. She/he could have a flower in her/his room and/or on the dinner tray. How about a badge to wear? It can be passed from one resident of the week to the next and should be easily recognized by residents and staff so that everyone knows that this person is royalty for the week and should be treated accordingly. By the end of the week we should have a beaming person who thinks she/he is great!

Community Action

It surely helps our self esteem if we feel we have some influence. The opposite is also true. Our self esteem is lessened when we feel that there is nothing we can do about the things we think are wrong.

To give the residents a feeling of power and to help them develop ideas that energize them hold a community action class or forum. Give them assistance with writing letters to the editor, the governor, their senators and representatives, not to mention the administration of the nursing home, businesses, Social Security, the president, or anybody or anyplace where they think change is needed or they have a comment or suggestion to make. In most instances they will get a reply. This can be shared with the group. Even if nothing is changed, the fact that someone took notice of their concerns will give them a high.

Ms. TS went on a group outing with five other residents. They planned a restaurant lunch. It was an event they cherished, but were disappointed when the advertised dessert of the day was not available to them because the restaurateur had run out. Ms. TS took the matter up with the community action group. A letter was written. The entire group received vouchers for a free dessert of their choice at the restaurant. The elation at this victory carried the group for weeks. They felt so good about themselves.

Mr. SR was almost run down by a youngster on a skateboard when he went with a group to a local shopping center. He was badly shaken, but not hurt. His fright turned to anger that ruined his outing. A call to the zoning board and a letter to the editor started action. Mr. SR was thrilled to read the newspaper account of skateboarders being apprehended and their activities curtailed. A special feeling of pride assailed him on his next incident free visit to the shopping center.

Letters and calls of complaint are not the only action a united group can take. They can also send out letters of appreciation and commendation to organizations and individuals to express pleasure and thanks. They will have the opportunity to let them know why they approve. It feels stupendous to have our complaints considered. Equally great is the feeling that our approbation has meaning to others.

Current Events

Many nursing home residents do not keep up with the news because of problems with hearing or sight. As they fall behind it all becomes more and more mind boggling as there is more and more information to process. They lose interest in current events. Consequently, they are lost in many conversations that go on around them and miss out on one avenue of communication they might have with their families and friends. It lowers self esteem to appear confused or befuddled about what is going on in the world, the country, the community. A group on newsworthy items that brings them up to date while drawing on their knowledge of history as they lived it is effective in maintaining self esteem and giving them a feeling of mastery. If the news involves a country ask them where their ancestors came from. Find out what they know about that country and slowly bring them to the present with what is happening in that area. If the reports are on a current scandal regarding money, the federal government, big business, or sports figures draw on their knowledge of what occurred on that topic in the past and tie it in with the present. They all know of similar outrageous events in the past that can be compared with what is happening now. Use maps, diagrams, a chalkboard, or videos to refresh their memory. Make it entertaining and make the residents do part of the teaching by giving the historical perspective. They'll be impressed with their own knowledge and delighted to be able to put it to use.

Celebrations

Celebrate all special events in the residents' lives, but have more lavish celebrations for the more significant milestones. Let the residents know that they are tops for having achieved something quite rare such as turning ninety years old! Any birthday is important as it is the resident's own day. There is no such thing as too much attention when there is a good reason for it. Surely they deserve recognition for being born and being alive! It is fabulous to know that other people care enough to be happy for us on our birthdays. Jubilation, commemoration, and festivities in a person's honor enhances self esteem.

Visitors

Make sure that visitors sign in and include information as to whom they are visiting, what their relationship is and where they are from. Then at a specified time each day or week announce the above information. If it is not too unwieldy, put it in the newsletter or in some printed form. The actual announcement, when everyone is listening for it, such as at the beginning of a meal, sounds good to many of the residents. They find esteem in the fact that they had visitors, that they had many visitors, that a grandchild visited, or that someone came from far away to see them. If residents or staff inquire they then have the opportunity to explain why the person came to see them. They may find they know the same people. I became aware of how important this routine could be when I visited an alert, oriented, friend in a distant state. He insisted that I write down where I was from so this would be included when the visiting list was read. I was happy to oblige. This was a way that I, as a concerned friend, could bring some recognition to my acquaintance. It made me feel good that I could perform this act that made him feel better about himself.

Talent Shows

I would never be one to suggest that everybody has talent, but those who have it feel better about themselves when it is noticed, and those of us who know the talented, feel good that we know talented people who receive recognition. Somehow it makes us feel we are better because we associate with those who have an ability to entertain others. If you can find residents who can speak, dance, sing, play a musical instrument, or tell jokes, that is super. If they have relatives who can contribute in this way, wonderful. Don't forget the staff. Residents are thrilled to brag that their nursing assistant or their maintenance person sang a solo or played the piano. Inspire those with particular aptitudes to share their abilities and the spotlight. Once talent is displayed you may bring out some retiring people, who will observe, catch the enthusiasm, and muster up the courage to say, "I can do that."

Profiles

Monthly newsletters are great vehicles for catering to the residents' self esteem needs. Display a resident monthly, giving a short biography and reporting some interesting facts. After the specifics are compiled add information for the benefit of the residents' self esteem. Just the facts can be pretty dull. Try to fascinate the readers. We can say why friends and/or family have admired and appreciated the residents. We can include something about their excellent qualities that have appealed to the staff. Achievements, unusual occupations, hobbies, or places of residence should be included. Find the unique, the curious, the exceptional, and make the story reflect residents anybody would like to meet and know.

Pictures of Their Youth

Remember the game where each person brings a picture of themselves when they were young and then everyone else tries to guess who that person is? Make an all out effort to find the pictures of the residents when they were younger and play this game with them. Even if they can't guess they will have fun looking at the pictures and the residents will love hearing about what cute babies or handsome young persons they were.

In the residents' rooms display pictures of them as young adults. It adds a dimension and gives visitors an opportunity to remark on their good looks. Compliments are always good for self esteem.

Nostalgia Trips

When we have to give up something we enjoyed it is depressing, and it doesn't do much for our self esteem either. It feels like failure and deprivation. Alleviate this whenever possible by arranging for the residents to do the things they used to do. Plan outings to a ball game, go out to lunch, shop in the mall, see the decorations during the holidays, attend a club meeting, or go to the beach. The exhilaration of doing what they always enjoyed doing will make them feel more like independent human beings. Naturally, this raises their self esteem.

The Perfect Grandparents

Find the best grandmother and grandfather in the nursing home. But don't limit the qualifiers to two people. Pick out what you want in each and find the components to make the perfect person. Each grand- parent has many parts. List the parts and find the resident who has the ideal feature. You may want to use physical, emotional, social, and behavioral aspects to make the whole person. Consider selecting the best hair, cheeks, eyebrows, eyes, nose, eyelashes, lips, teeth, neck, shoulders, arms, hands, fingers, back, waist, stomach, chest, lap, legs, knees, ankles, feet, toes, grooming, clothes, nature, character, temperament, laugh, voice, smile, friend, listener.

The more best items we include the more residents we can mention and the more it will help self esteem.

Fashion Show

Fashion shows can be serious or funny or a combination. They can be contemporary or show clothes from past eras. Use the residents as models to show latest teenage fashions in comparison with styles worn in their youth. Models can be in wheelchairs or ambulatory. We can be silly or serious, displaying clothes for laughs or clothes appropriate for nursing home living.

Staff and family members can model. Everyone can share the limelight. Residents will be thrilled to be models, but will be equally pleased to see those they know appear before them. How about a hat show? Or we might consider theme fashion shows such as weddings, graduations, or children's school or Easter clothes. Grandchildren and children of staff members can be used for these last mentioned events. This will bring back happy memories. The residents will feel proud to be part of such extraordinary family events.

Groups for Learning

High School or College Classes

In our culture high status is awarded for education. The more schooling people have the more likely they are to be held in high esteem, other factors not considered. Besides, learning is stimulating and exciting. School is rewarding. When people do well they get immediate praise in the form of a good grade or acknowledgment of a correct answer.

Residents can go to the high school or the college for classes. If this is not feasible, most high schools and colleges offer off campus classes and can deliver them right to the nursing home. Classes can be geared to the students' interests and level of functioning.

As the residents gain knowledge, they gain esteem.

Skill Sharing

Most residents have some knowledge or ability they can pass on to others and feel better because they had something to give. Ms. RQ taught me how to clap in a way that enabled me to make real noise! Ms. QP explained how I could make persimmon pudding. Whenever I've had a particular problem with something they know about they've been able to solve it for me. At times they have volunteered unusual, but useful information such as how to crack a coconut or get into a pecan without smashing the nutmeat inside. These skills can be labeled with the resident's name as it is passed on from person to person or group to group. The tips can be compiled and printed in the newsletter or in a separate publication.

Whenever residents can do something better than another, have an original idea, or can teach a skill, use them and use their knowledge. They will feel better about themselves and develop an inner urge for further progress.

Health Education

It is ever so much less mysterious and more comfortable to have information and facts and know what is going on in our bodies. This decreases worry, stress, fear and the uncertainty regarding the motives of health care personnel. Set up classes on health problems for nursing home residents. They can be taught by professionals, but given in layman's terms so that the individual suffering from the disease can understand the symptoms, treatment, and prognosis. It feels good to have knowledge about what is happening to us and what we can do to help ourselves. The nagging guilt of not giving ourselves proper care can eat away at self esteem. Hearing that all that can be done is being done allows the individual to relax and get on with living.

Life Review

Life review classes are eminently useful for self esteem. As the residents' report on their lives they realize that they had worth, stature, excitement, happiness, and made a contribution to the world in which they lived. The satisfaction of sharing a commonalty and at the same time getting recognition for individual experiences is a heady affair.

Life review classes are excellent for enhancing the self esteem of those with poor short term memory because they will be able to talk fluently and comfortably about the past. They will love the fact that others want to listen to them and feel comforted that their memory is good for some things.

Trivia

Trivia games are popular because they are good for people's self esteem. We feel smart when we can answer questions that show off our knowledge of little known facts - information that would be difficult to work into a normal conversation. Only through trivia games can we discuss these unimportant, but fascinating trifles. The nursing home residents enjoy trivia too. They also like to dredge up filed away information and think about old time radio, old songs, sports figures, cars, rhymes, fairy tales, movies, and stars of days gone by. They can exercise their minds, flaunt their intelligence, have some fine memories, and augment their esteem while they are at it!

Craft Groups

What is amazing is the number of people who do not have artistic talent, or have not developed it beyond the kindergarten level. Since so many of us share the same lack of skill in crafts this limitation need not keep anyone from participating in craft groups and experiencing the esteem that comes from creating something.

Let those who know how to make things teach others so they can devise decorations for the facility, for their own room, or to give to friends and relatives. Preparing artifacts for the times the nursing home is decorated for holidays lets the residents know that they are needed for their contributions and that what they do is worthy of display. Handmade decorations in their own rooms are always conversation openers with the residents getting admiration for what they have done. It feels good for them to be able to give away something that they have made with their own hands.

Self Improvement Groups

Relaxation Groups

Stress doesn't lessen with age. Stressors may change, but there is always stress. Staff can do some things to relieve the nursing home residents' stress by controlling the environment and giving good care. However, most people's stress can only be controlled by themselves.

Most stress comes from inside ourselves, rather than from external factors. It is how we interpret the event, rather than the event itself, that causes stress. We can learn how to control stress. There are many techniques. One is relaxation. There are many ways to relax. They all work for someone. Try several and have the residents pick the ones that are right for them. We can teach relaxation techniques ranging from progressive relaxation, to guided imagery, to thought replacement, to visualization, to relaxing to music. Descriptions of the methods follow.

Relaxation

1. In a quiet environment, have the residents sit in a comfortable position.
2. Instruct them to close their eyes.
3. Have them deeply relax all their muscles, beginning at the feet and progressing to the face.
4. Tell the residents to breathe through their nose and concentrate on their breath as they breathe out.

5. The residents should continue this for several minutes and then sit quietly for several more minutes before opening their eyes.

Guided Imagery

Take the residents on an imaginary trip in which the leader is the director of the tour.

1. Have the residents close their eyes.
2. Describe the following scenario step by step.
    a. Imagine that you are leaving the facility.
    b. You are leaving your cares and troubles behind.
    c. You are crossing a bridge and moving towards a sloping hill.
    d. You approach the hill.
    e. You are going up a winding path.
    f. There is a place to stop along the path and you sit and rest for awhile.
    g. You take some time to examine the tension in your body and the stress in your life.
    h. You take all your stresses and tensions and put them down on the side of the path.
    i. Leaving the tensions and stresses behind, you feel freer and lighter and you continue on the path to the top of the hill.
    j. You look down at the river in the valley.
    k. What do you see?
    l. Take in all your surroundings. What do you hear? What do you smell? This is your special place. You are relaxed and comfortable in this place.

m. This is your own special place and you can go to this place to relax whenever you want.

n. Come back to the room, but realize that the place where you were was your own place that you created. You can use it whenever you want to feel relaxed.

We can use this or any other series of instructions that are interesting, comforting, and enjoyable.

Thought Replacement

In thought replacement we take negative thoughts and help the residents turn them into positive ones. We teach them how to stop their worries and fears and think success and ability. The group can practice together. Once they have a positive script, they should write it down so that they can refer to it whenever they feel under stress or are in a situation where their negative thoughts are dominant. We can call the group the positive thinking group. We begin by listing all their worries and fears and then giving them positive sayings and pleasant suggestions to take their place. The group should meet regularly to reinforce their positive statements. Since our everyday life is full of sayings that hold promise that everything will be all right, they will be able to contribute many. Some we might use are:

Everything is for the best.

I can handle that.

It will be all right.

It will soon be over.

I can do it.

Worry doesn't help.

There is nothing to worry about.

I'll take it step by step.

I will have help.

There is nothing to fear.

Mistakes won't hurt.

I can relax.

I don't have to get tense.

This will end.

I've survived worse.

Teach the residents to make these statements to themselves whenever they feel nervous.

Ms. PO always worried that her daughter would have an accident whenever she went away on any sort of a trip. She went to the support group and expressed her fears. She was assured that worry would not do anything but make her uncomfortable. With group support she decided that whenever she started to feel nervous about her daughter she would think instead that her daughter was a good and safe driver and that everything would be all right. She practiced very hard by herself and with the group members. She was able to let her worrying trigger the reassuring thought. Soon she was able to drive the fear from her mind.

Visualization

In visualization both tension and relaxation are visualized as objects. The exercise goes like this.

1. Have the residents close their eyes.
2. Ask the residents to be aware of the tensions in their bodies and the worries in their minds.
3. Have the residents visualize all their tensions and pains as ice.

4. Tell the residents to visualize the feeling of relaxation as the sun.
5. The residents can now visualize the sun melting the ice – the relaxation driving out the tensions.

Other symbols that might be used are fire-water, cereal-spoon, dark-light, or colors, such as red to blue.

Listening to Music

Music can be very relaxing to people who lose themselves in it. One half hour of music is about right for a relaxation session. It must be music that is pleasing, soothing, and agreeable to the residents' tastes.

To relax to music the residents should get comfortable, close their eyes, scan their bodies for tension, and then concentrate on the music. If any unrelated thought creeps into their minds, they may be told to note it, discard it, and go back to listening to the music. When the music stops they can again scan their bodies for tension and see if there is any difference from when they started the exercise.

The residents who learn this skill will feel better physically and mentally. Better health means better self esteem.

Relationship Groups

A group can be set up just to deal with relationships and social outreach. In this group the residents can be given the opportunity to learn how to get along with each other and reach out to others in the facility. The group concentrates on social support. The residents are assigned outreach tasks geared towards enhancing their self esteem. They try out each assigned social skill in the group and then perform it with other residents in the nursing home.

Some suggested social skills are:

1. Find someone in this group you do not know out two interesting facts about her/him. Share two facts about yourself. Now do this with another resident in the facility.

2. Identify someone you like in the group. Tell her/him you like her/him. Do the same with someone you know in the facility.

3. Find someone you think you can trust and tell her/him something that makes you proud of yourself. Then share your greatest worry with her/him. Do this same exercise with another resident who does not come to the group.

4. As tactfully as you can, make a suggestion to someone that would help her/him be a better person. Perhaps it will have something to do with the way she/he talks, acts, dresses. Perform this same task outside the group.

5. Tell someone in the group what you admire about her/him. Now tell another facility resident what you admire about her/him.

6. Tell someone in the group what you plan to do to improve yourself. Find someone outside the group to share this with too.

Different tasks can be assigned at each weekly meeting. Some tasks can be repeated. Always praise and rejoice in the residents' successes.

As the residents learn to handle themselves socially and as they see how their attentions to others are welcomed they will become more and more confident in the way they manage themselves in the company of others. They will feel liked and likable.

Recognition Groups

A major social skill is small talk. Those who don't do it well generally hate parties and meeting new people. Living in a nursing home necessitates the meeting of many new people. The ability to handle it well promotes self esteem. Most small talk conversations start with the weather and progress to where the person lives. Anything beyond that constitutes a more prolonged engagement and actually getting to know the person. In a recognition group the residents will learn to feel good about their social acumen. Also, they will meet people who have qualities in common with them. This kind of recognition never fails to make us feel good. In a recognition group certain people can be specified for distinction, which further benefits their self esteem. Let me explain.

1. Recognizing new people in the group. The social skills involved in successfully recognizing new people are knowing how to be friendly and obtaining basic information such as where they are from and when they arrived. We can model this skill for the residents or set up a procedure so that each takes a turn in welcoming the new person or persons.

2. Recognizing things in common. Use the group as a vehicle for each member to find someone with something in common with her/him. This can be played as a game. Each participant sets out to find others with certain characteristics. Each person is given a list of five items, such as a mutual friend, from the same place, the same number of children, the same age, the same job when working, etc. There is no end to this type of scavenger hunt. It can be done in one place or with the residents sent out into the nursing home to locate people with similarities. It is fun. It leads to discovery. It develops friendships. Most importantly, it reinforces the resident's sense of self.

3. Recognizing differences. Play the same game, but ask the resident to find the person who has different color eyes than she/he has, is taller or shorter, has no grandchildren if she/he has many, lived out of the country if she/he has never left the state, or loves animals if she/he doesn't. Let them find that they are unique and that their uniqueness is valuable and interesting.

4. Recognizing individuals. Let the group members find the individuals who are the oldest, the youngest, the tallest, the shortest, from the farthest away, have the most children, were married the longest, have the most hair, have the least hair, had the most jobs, had the most interesting jobs. This will take some research, maybe some debate. It will be stimulating. The reward is self esteem.

Extra Strokes Group

There are residents who do not know how to get the attention they crave. Bring them to a daily social group. Give them a welcome. Cater to them. Feed them goodies. Smile and enjoy them. Listen to them. Pat and praise them. When possible, solve their problems. Have as much staff as possible present to be attentive to them. These extra strokes will bring them great satisfaction. Being singled out and given attention for a short period of time each day will enable them to feel good, increase their self esteem, and elevate their mood.

Form a group to reach out to the residents who need extra strokes. Meet regularly with residents who will each be assigned a resident to cherish. They will be expected to regularly contact the resident. Instructions will be given for meeting individual needs and weekly projects will be explained. Weekly projects can include listening to music together, eating together, giving a gift, understanding a need, working on communication, playing a game, decorating the bed side stand, or any number of simple attentions. The weekly meetings also serve as a place to report progress, tell anecdotal information, and give praise and inspiration. The residents receiving the attention flourish and exhibit more responsive and pleasant personalities. The residents giving the time and care do well too because they can see that their work is meaningful. Their self esteem is helped while they help others. Usually a real bond is made between the resident giver and the resident receiver. Sometimes it is hard to tell who is getting the most out of the relationship.

Mr. ON was a demanding resident who always wanted more. One week into his Extra Strokes group his rate of wanting and the intensity of his requests was noticeably down. His only major demand seemed to be that he be taken to the group on time. There he got to make all his complaints, knew he was heard, and got extra coddling besides. This decreased his anxiety and raised his comfort level.

Ms. NM was an Extra Strokes provider. She was assigned Ms. ML. No one really liked Ms. ML as her standard response to everything was "No." Ms. NM was determined to carry out her assignment, was reinforced in her efforts in the weekly meeting, and started to get quite attached to Ms. ML as she invested her energy and care in her. Slowly Ms. ML began to trust her Extra Stroker and was much more positive in her outlook and response. Ms. NM had her success recognized. She made a friend in the process.

Confidentiality continues to be crucial. When incidents are shared, names must never be used. Identifying information is not disclosed in the group.

Teach Self Appreciation

Strength Groups

Have group members identify one nice thing about themselves and one nice thing about each member in the group. Each day group members add one more item to the list so that when the group meets the next week they have a long list of good things about themselves.

The group members give each member another compliment, which they add to their list, and for another week they write down one more accomplishment or pleasure. The third week finds them with a longer list of heart warming positives about themselves. Have this small group continue for three weeks, then start with another, retaining one or two of the former group to teach the new group.

It is uncomfortable for most of us to hear compliments and praise about ourselves as we are more accustomed to modesty and criticism. Nevertheless, dwelling on our own goodness can bring on a gleam that generates strength and well being. Overcoming the initial reluctance to do this is not easy. Sometimes it is best to start with some simple exercise such as having each resident hug and pat themselves on the back in self appreciation and self love. From there it can be explained that it is important to like ourselves so that we can like others. Then, instead of going directly into the announcement of what they like about themselves they can say what they like about others in the room.

Since we are so unused to setting down our own good qualities, examples and choices may need to be given to the residents. Have them think about personal qualities, temperament, looks, accomplishments, abilities, pleasures, and possessions. Some strengths they might consider are: accepting, admirable, ambitious, artistic, attractive, aware, busy, capable, careful, charming, convincing, dignified, distinctive, efficient, energetic, expressive, friendly, full of ideas, gentle, gogetter, individualistic, kind, leader, likes new ideas, looked up to, loyal, manager, motivated, musical, neat, open-minded, orderly, overcoming, poised, pursuing, reliable, respected, searching, self determining, sharp, spontaneous, stable, steadfast, steady, strong-willed, systematic, tactful, thinker, thoughtful, tireless, trusting, trustworthy, understanding, unselfish, vivacious, well-informed, witty.

This list is comprised of personal qualities. We can make additional lists in other categories such as appearance, accomplishments, abilities, and pleasures.

For example:

Appearance: Athletic, beautiful, cute, delightful demeanor, exciting lips, flawless complexion, good shape, high cheek bones, interesting looks, jovial appearance, kind eyes, lovely, many expressions, nice skin, outstanding hair, pleasant expression, quick movements, rich looking clothes, slim, tastefully dressed, usually smiling, vigorous, winsome, youthful, zestful.

Accomplishments and Abilities: Awards for service, ball player, can add numbers in head, directed office staff, earned a living, farmed, gave to charity, had children, invented something, jitter-bugged, kept the family records, loved the family, married, needleworker, organized the women's/men's club, played the piano, quilter, restored furniture, sky-diver, taught, understood foreign languages, voted, walked to school, yachter.

Pleasures: Activities, ball games, cards, desserts, evenings, eating, friends, games, health, joking, kidding, laughing, music, needlework, outings, parties, reading, snapshots, sleeping, sports, television, visiting, writing.

Dream Groups

It has been said that when we stop dreaming, we are dead. This is, no doubt, an extreme statement. Nevertheless, our dreams are important to us. As long as we have dreams, we have hope. Hope is essential to on-going life. As children we may have been accused of day dreaming too much, but our day dreaming served a useful purpose for us. Through day dreams we were charting what we wanted in our life and rehearsing how we would make it happen, or how we would handle it when it did happen. Dreams can help the elderly prepare in the same way. It can be called preparation, or rehearsal, or we can make it more romantic and call it dreaming.

Residents can dream about what they want to happen in their lives and then dream about how they will bring it about. An example of this would be Ms. LK's wish that her husband would visit in the evening instead of the afternoon. He came one time a day, and always during an activity she particularly enjoyed. She did not know how to ask him to adjust his visiting time to her schedule, thinking his time was so much more valuable than hers. She didn't want to offend him or let him think that she didn't prize his visits. She dreamed of what she wanted and dreamed of a way to confront him with the problem. She dreamed she was successful and in actuality was able to accomplish the task in a tactful way and achieve the wanted result.

Several residents may have a group dream such as a desire to attend a certain event, change something in the facility, or manage a part of their lives. As a group they can dream of the event and see themselves doing as they want. As they imagine themselves accomplishing what they want they can come up with many alternatives to get the outcome they want. They can find encouragement and solutions in their mutual dream.

This technique helps the residents learn problem solving. They can picture the desired conclusion and then move to fulfill it. It will give them a feeling of being less at the mercy of others. It will give them hope. It will give them self esteem.

Looking Good Groups

Look better, feel better, have more confidence. It all goes together. Any groups geared to improved physical appearance pay off in increased self esteem. We have noticed that the beauty operator in the nursing home is always busy. The residents with the new hair-dos act more sprightly and proud. Set up groups that deal solely with appearance. Have groups that make it possible for the residents to learn about style, the latest colors, trends, and fashions. Let them fool around with make-up, manicures, and hair styles. They'll love the attention and blossom with self esteem.

Self Discovery Games

Simple, unscientific methods that enable us to focus on ourselves are fun and good for self esteem. This partly explains the popularity of fortune tellers, palm readers, and horoscopes. The idea is to concentrate on the good and positive areas. The residents enjoy the pleasant focus of attention and get a kick out of the element of mystery and revelation.

Any number of pop psychology questionnaires from current magazines or books may be used as long as the results are light and flattering. Fortune cookies even work for the purposes of this group. The residents will abstract their own truths, dismiss the far fetched, think about the predictions and pronouncements, and go away with a glow.

We can devise self exploration games such as personality traits and favorite colors. If the most liked color is yellow they are sunny, optimistic, cheerful. The blues are calming, serene comforting. Reds are vibrant, outgoing. Purples love people. Anyway, the notion is to enjoy, stimulate, and give esteem.

A FEW LAST WORDS

In all exercises the stress is on giving residents a feeling of usefulness and recognition not authority and supremacy. Guard against the residents assuming too much power. Although this may be good for their self esteem, it would not be good for the self esteem of their peers.

By now I hope we will have said to ourselves that we already do everything mentioned in this book. Good for us! It is all just part of doing a good job. We should have high self esteem for performing so well at work and enhancing the self esteem of others.

We also realize that we do not magically raise another person's self esteem, nor is there one important and crucial move we can make to improve self esteem. We see that it is a combination of many small, on going attitudes and actions. We don't make the residents feel good about themselves. We set the stage so that they can develop their own feelings of high self esteem. We do everything we can to allow this to happen!

THE END

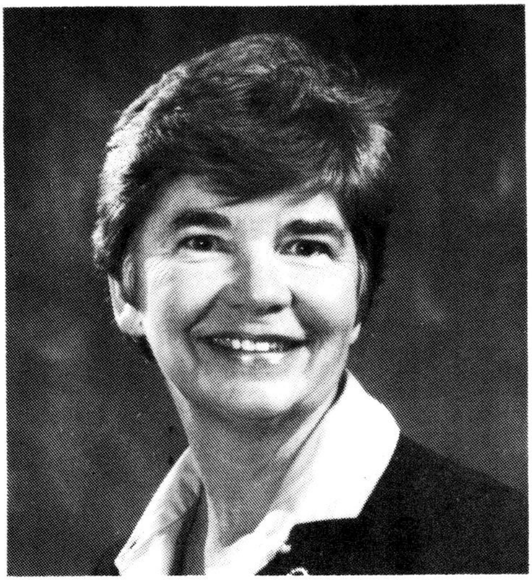

Dr. Marylou Hughes has been involved in the field of gerontology not only as a consultant and provider of inservice training to nursing home staff, but as a teacher, administrator, psychotherapist, and writer. She has worked with the elderly in mental health, institutional, rehabilitation, home and state settings.

Include in Dr. Hughes' background are experiences in children's services, crisis intervention, and program development. For the past twenty plus years she has worked in social services as an employee of the Department of Health and Rehabilitation Services in Florida, and later in rehabilitation and mental health centers and hospitals. She is currently self-employed as a marriage counselor, psychotherapist, teacher and consultant to several private facilities in Florida.

Other books written by Dr. Hughes: *The Nursing Home and the Resident's Relatives*; *Mental Health Problems and the Nursing Home Resident*; *Revised Social Service Care Plans for Long Term Care Facilities; Restorative Approach for Nursing Home Social Workers; Social Service Policies & Procedures for LTC Facilities; Essential Psychosocial Inservices for Nursing Home Personnel; Inservices on Loss, Families, and Aging; Dying, Death, and Loss in Long-Term Care; Group Psychotherapy in Long-Term Care; Individual Psychotherapy in Long-Term Care Settings; The Long-Term Care Family Manual*

Enhancing The Self-Esteem
of The Nursing Home Resident
ISBN 1-877735-16-7
9 781877 735165